AS LONG AS YOU SING, I'LL DANCE

AS LONG AS YOU SING, I'LL DANCE

*The bond not the burden –
the blessing of reciprocal caregiving*

JULIA SOTO LEBENTRITT

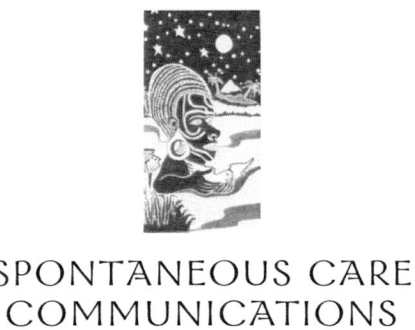

SPONTANEOUS CARE
COMMUNICATIONS

As Long as You Sing, I'll Dance:
The bond not the burden – the blessing of reciprocal caregiving

Copyright © 2012 by Julia Soto Lebentritt

All rights reserved. No part of this book may be used or reproduced in any form, electronic or mechanical, including photocopying, recording, or scanning into any information storage and retrieval system, without written permission from the author except in the case of brief quotation embodied in critical articles and reviews.

This book is based on Julia Soto Lebentritt's experiences over a 40-year period. Names have been changed, characters combined and events compressed. Certain episodes are imaginative recreation, and those episodes are not intended to portray actual events.

Illustrations in the book:	Art by Jeanne A. Benas • www.BenasArt.com
Cover design/artwork:	Armando Soto • www.armansoto.com Including "Taino Images of the Caribbean," "Ancient Greek Dancer" and "Safety of Passage"
	Jeanne A. Benas • www.BenasArt.com "Garden Party Dance Circle"
Book Design:	Melissa Mykal Batalin • www.thetroybookmakers.com Using Palatino and Gill Sans Std.
Author Photo:	Natalie Cartz • www.NatalieCartzPhotography.com
Publisher:	Spontaneous Care Communications, DBA Troy, New York
Editing:	Rob Brill
Book orders:	Spontaneous Care Communications, DBA P.O. Box 1357 • Troy, NY 12181-1357 Email: julia@reciprocalcare.com Online at tbmbooks.com or amazon.com
ISBN:	978-1-61468-072-7

Dedication to Caregivers

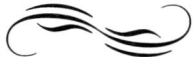

Long before I started my work with the elderly, I experienced a staggering personal loss with my own mother.

In 1984, while visiting my aging parents in Troy, New York, I came into the kitchen from a walk around the old neighborhood. My mother turned from doing dishes. "I've been meaning to tell you," she said, "I am wondering who you are anyway?" She began to question me in a hostile way. This was the first time that my mother ever told me that she didn't know me and I was not her daughter. I argued with her and told her she was wrong.

The second night after she first disclosed her confusion, I was standing in the kitchen alone drinking water at the sink. In her nightgown, robe and slippers, she shuffled by me through the kitchen down the short flight of stairs to lock the back door. Then she said very loudly, "10:45! It's time to go to bed!"

I was gazing at the beautiful full moon. I could see her stop and look at me in the window reflection. When I turned to see what she wanted and why she stopped to stare at me, I said something like "Drinking some water, I'll go to bed soon…."

Given her response, "Are you whispering or talking out loud?" I knew that she had taken her hearing aide out so I repeated myself louder. Then she smiled meaningfully (as if she had caught me doing something wrong) and walked away toward her bedroom. I thought has she seen my mind? I felt I was being kicked out of my childhood home. She needed help, and so did I.

I realized then that she was in the early stages of Alzheimer's disease. It was not long before my mother became impossible to reach. I honestly thought it was due to three things: her hearing loss, her memory loss and most of all her willful decision to withdraw her love from me and the family.

The pain of not being able to relate to someone's dementia causes staggering anger, depression and isolation. My mother's cognitive changes over the next few years would continue to cause a chaos of negative feelings and beliefs among her caregivers and family and friends.

We were lonely when she no longer played her traditional roles as our mother and our father's wife. Mornings, Daddy would find her sitting half-dressed at the kitchen table waiting. No hot coffee or breakfast juice and cereals ready on the table. Their roles reversed. We felt abandoned and burdened by what used to be her unsung daily chores.

As her personal caregiver my father was angry at her and could never understand that something organic was happening inside her body. He dismissed her strange behaviors saying, "She always was a lazy girl." In fact she always was a hard working mom of four children. Now there was a mounting turmoil in our parents' home and relationship.

When she grabbed her pocketbook and tried to leave the house, my father fought with her at the back door. She fought back and escaped. Instead of calling his nearby sons, my father called the police. They found her at her best friend's house two doors away visiting and sipping tea.

She fell and broke her wrist ending up in a bed in the front room next to the TV. We all came home to debate what could be done. There was guilt among some of us and additional caregiving for others. She cried easily and called and wrote ragged half-sentence apologies for her confusion and mistakes.

Now more and more people are caregiving for elders with dementia and suffering the same emotional, physical and spiritual burdens. When Margaret M. Kelly read the following poem at a hospice Remembrance Service recently, I heard my mother's and my family's story again.

"Hailstorm in Her Mind"
by Margaret M. Kelly

In Memory of Margaret Ashman Kelly
2/26/25–5/9/10

It's hailing thoughts in my mother's mind –
The hailstones fly about wildly.

She reaches out to catch them:
    "Where is…"
    "Let's talk about…"
    "What should we do…"
    "We should think about…"
But each time the hail stone melts too soon.

I'm out in the storm, too,
Trying to catch a few for her.
I used to be able to finish her sentences for her,
But now the hailstones I catch for her,
Melt too soon in the warm hands of my concern.

I am also rendered speechless
And, like my mother, just sit in silence.

I am reduced to giving hugs and caresses
To a woman who never liked to be touched.

But I can't give her hailstones anymore.

As I listened to Margaret's powerful poem I thought – here is another daughter suffering like I did. Later I found out that our mothers' lives and roles as women in the world were extremely different. Margaret's mother had a professional career in education and journalism whereas my mom, Marcella Gontier Lebentritt, completed 6th grade, worked in a shirt factory and became a stay-at-home mom. This illustrates the universality of Alzheimer's disease. As we know, presidents or laborers, male or female at almost any age can become victims.

Margaret's words – "You are killing BOTH of us," from another poem titled "I Hate You, Alzheimer's" express so well the desperation of caregiving for the cognitively impaired. I want to thank her for letting me share her thoughts about how insanely tough it is to care for a loved one who has cognitive loss.

Can caregiving really be better than you think? Can you enjoy being a professional or non-professional caregiver? Can you relax using song and caregiving traditions?

This book is dedicated to caregivers who struggle – and hopefully can develop the skills – to relate to those for whom they care.

Julia Soto Lebentritt

Contents

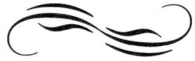

About the Title xiii
Introduction *by Christine Knowles, RN, BC* xv
Preface for Caregiving and Caregivers xix

Part 1: Following the Thread of Our Mothers' Joyful Caregiving

1. When you're a caregiver,
   you're passing on the legacy of caregiving. 3
   It seems we could never forget these caregiving ways…
   An elder pleads for gentle caregiving
   Don't *baby* me! Just take care of me with kindness

2. When you are a spontaneous caregiver,
   you are in a happily developing relationship 13
   Two examples of spontaneous caregiving relationships

3. Caring is about something much larger than caregiving 18
   Illustration: The Problem

4. Care about what they care about 23

5. Your spontaneous powers 26
   Listen, Feel more, See more, Be aware, Be more alive,
   Walk in their shoes, Accommodate, Be playful,
   Reclaim your voice, And affirm…

6. Free up your spontaneous powers quiz 38

Part 2: Rhythmic Movements and Spontaneous Songs

7. Conducting: The leader's communication to performers. . . . 45
   The five-week-old conductor
   Leader's Guide: Get everyone gently moving
   The wheelchair conductors
   Coaching spirits

8. Spontaneous songs: The ordinary instinct of birds singing. . . 50
   Sisters' duet
   Leader's Guide: Rhythm sharing
   Elders' duets
   Coaching spirits

9. Greetings: Familiar calls from long ago. 56
   Bedtime calls
   Leader's Guide: Lullabies with childhood memories
   Remembering childhood calls
   Coaching spirits

10. Humming: Meaningful murmurs of living. 61
    The humming mother and mosquitoes
    Leader's Guide: Something everyone can do!
    Mmmmmmmm – they're all thoughts
    Coaching spirits

11. Communications of love:
    Touching is language is singing is dancing. 69
    Simple human touch
    Leader's Guide: Soothe! soothe! soothe!
    Connecting the eyes with the ears and the skin
    Coaching spirits

12. Patterns of light, sound, motion:
    The breathing presence of energy that connects us 73
    Lois's colors
    Leader's Guide: Chanting lulling syllables
    The magic of imagination
    Coaching spirits

13. There's rhythm everywhere:
    Sharpen your personal communication style with gestures . . 79
    "La linda manita"
    Leader's Guide: Harriet the monkey
    Max the cat visits
    Coaching spirits

Part 3: Traditions

14. Participatory chant: The comfort of a storytelling circle 91
    A story of creation
    Leader's Guide: Aloha greeting
    "Down by the butternut tree"
    Coaching spirits

15. Praising with familiar kind words: The warmth of words . . . 98
    My carnation
    Leader's Guide: Praise songs
    Make every hour sweet as a flower
    Coaching spirits

16. Lullaby memories: Bewitching tales of the past 102
    A Greek mother
    Leader's Guide: Storytellers
    The first time she felt loved
    Coaching spirits

17. Sing the blues: Bonding with cries 108
    In the beginning, there was the blues
    Leader's Guide: Memorials that evoke emotions
    Honoring diversity
    Coaching spirits

18. Following traditions: Positive feelings of
    old sheets and vintage tunes. 114
    Sounds and smells that soothe
    Leader's Guide: Harvest sensory treasures
    Gershwin tunes
    Coaching spirits

19. Power songs and prayers:
    The soulful opportunities of traditions 121
        Nurturing moonlit memories
        Leader's Guide: Simple songs
        Nursery rhymes
        "Hush Little Baby"
        "Kumbaya"
        "Starlight, Star Bright"
        Sharing prayers
        Sundowning
        Coaching spirits

20. Finding home in lullabies:
    The longing for someone somewhere. 131
        In the beginning, there was mother and home
        Leader's Guide: Going home
        "Home, Home on the Range"
        Coaching spirits

CODA: The "bye-bye" in lullabies. .137

Acknowledgements 141

Julia's Spontaneous Life 145

NOTES 151

About the Title
As Long as You Sing, I'll Dance:
The bond not the burden—
the blessing of reciprocal caregiving

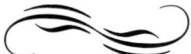

A cherished caregiving moment from the end of a long day inspires the title:

The first babbling of Angelina's voice sprang from her connection to "Row, Row, Row Your Boat." She and I sang "row, row, row" over and over and over while others repeated the round.

As time went by, Angelina burst into songs without words – nonsense sounds, riffs, jazz scats, refrains containing a multitude of lulling and playful sounds in many languages, human and animal voices – do de da and gushing contagious laughter.

Next, I challenged her: "Angelina, as long as you sing, I'll dance." We performed a long duet, and I knew she could hear and control us with her voice and will power.

Her vibrant dark eyes flickered like burning coals. Weighing 60 pounds, 90-plus years old, nodding yes, shaking her chin no, Angelina now made her needs and desires known. Musical communications helped staff members understand that she could and would declare her independence, reinstating her inalienable rights as a person.

When I first said "As long as you sing, I'll dance" to Angelina, I meant "As long as you breathe, I'll wash the dishes, cook, and go to work, shop, and come home and bathe you and me, as if I am always dancing."

Pete Seeger wrote a bedtime story about a fearsome monster based on a South African lullaby and folk story. A little boy and his father are inspired to sing the monster's name, Abiyoyo, as a hypnotic song. The rhythm affects Abiyoyo and forces him to dance and gradually fall down fast asleep. Caregivers can quiet their own inner monsters as well as give quality care by using the charms of lullabies.

Lao-tzu wrote in Chapter 11 of the Tao:
> We join spokes together in a wheel
> But it is the center hole
> That makes the wagon move.

Throughout my life I have met many amazing unique individuals who were receptive to my work. Among them, Christine Knowles who understood my approach and helped me name the method of caregiving I am teaching, Reciprocal Caregiving.

The mother's heartbeat is at the core of Reciprocal Caregiving. The universal pattern of the heartbeat is a rhythm found in the music of the world. Before medications, surgeries and other invasive medical approaches, in many cultures the drum and heartbeat rhythm were used to heal. In *Silent Pulse*, author George Leonard calls this rhythm the "silent pulse" that "connects us to every thing in the universe."

Reciprocal Caregiving involves us in finding similarity and likeness – mutual response – interchange like one drummer calls to another resulting in unity and oneness. Spontaneity is at the heart of the caregiver who trades evenly, exchanges, gives and takes, heartbeat for heartbeat.

Introduction
By Christine Knowles, RN, BC

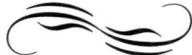

Human beings exhibit many remarkable abilities like the use of language and the capacity to create and appreciate beauty. We draw upon an amazing complex of emotional states and a concept of self and "others." We also possess less enviable traits, such as an appetite for violence, selfishness and greed. When those we love lose the very cognitive principle that animates us and sets us apart as humans we realize we possess another skill, a most divine gift within us – the power to comfort and soothe.

In *As Long as You Sing, I'll Dance,* Julia Soto Lebentritt enlightens us on this deep and almost mystical ability to comfort others. Her book is part history, part healthcare, part training manual and a comprehensive instruction on how to help heal our own hearts while caretaking others.

Julia has masterfully woven a tapestry of stories that illustrate both with the written word and with an optional accompanying CD the power of the human voice to calm the agitated mind. She reveals how to use the tool of healing touch for elders who are starved for it; the strength of eye contact to reach into a frightened soul and steady it; the magic of a smile that blows away the clouds of dementia's cold grip. Her book describes a toolbox of caretaking skills that we humans have learned over the centuries, paramount being the voice of comfort.

That voice is described through Julia's fascinating analysis of lullabies. She explores their association with communicating to the distressed, whether a tiny baby crying or a confused elderly dementia patient. We see how the lullaby has come full circle. "As Long as You Sing, I'll Dance" details that evolution and how we can use it to impact the lives of our loved ones stricken with dementia as well as our selves, worn-out and down by the burden of caretaking.

My earliest and favorite memory of my mother was her rocking me in her little white rocking chair singing "Too-ra-loora-loora." When she was deeply into her dementia, I used to sit by her and hold her hand singing that same song. She often called me "Mama" then. My mother's lullaby became her own healing modality through me. The skill of comforting passed down from mother to daughter.

My sisters and I were with my mother as she died. We sat around her bed holding her and each other's hands. I brought in a CD player and played all of her favorite Irish songs while my sisters and I sang along. It was as much for our comfort as for hers. A part of me died that day along with her. The child, the daughter, the one who was nurtured and loved unconditionally no longer had that safe harbor. But the privilege of having provided my mother a "safe passage and a good death" helped to heal my loss.

In her book Julia teaches us how to employ those very skills of comforting that we learned from our loved ones and to use them as a way to communicate with those who have been silenced by Alzheimer's or dementia. She provides us with guideposts as we walk through that dark forest that can help us regain some semblance of relationship with loved ones we may have thought we could no longer know. By teaching us how to care take, Julia teaches us how to feel loved once again.

In this country and around the world we are facing a dramatic increase in Alzheimer's disease and other forms of dementia. Populations are aging and healthcare is trying to adapt to accommodate this new paradigm. The old model of psychiatric nursing being the primary field for nurses' caretaking those who have disabilities of the mind has branched out. Now the specialty of geriatric nursing is helping to define the treatment and plan of care for our elderly dementia patients. With this shift in focus we need to develop innovative models of care that incorporate all the players on the stage: patient, loved one, physician, nurse and Certified Nursing Assistant.

In over 25 years in the field of psychiatric nursing and human services, I have never come across a plan of caring for both the patient and the caretaker as beautifully integrated as is found here. This book can revolutionize the way we approach dementia patients. It can also provide a necessary lifeline of knowledge to those who care for them, in facilities as well as at home.

We all come into this world needing comfort, and we all leave with the same need. "As Long as You Sing, I'll Dance "is the lullaby we can use to fill that need.

PREFACE
For Caregiving and Caregivers

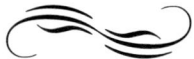

Life coach and best-selling author Dan Miller talks about "approaching the usual in an unusual way."

I invite you here to hold opposites together in your mind – the caregiving new mother and the geriatric nurse; the newborn baby and the old woman or man needing your assistance; the plan of care and the infinite creativity inherent in our daily duties and minds. As you view your work in these opposite ways, Miller writes in *No More Dreaded Mondays*, "you will suspend your normal thinking process and allow an intelligence beyond rational thought to create new solutions." May this book about care and connection make your caregiving more meaningful and help you feel more comfortable and open toward one another.

A mother winds the key on the mobile over her daughter's crib and "Raindrops Keep Falling on My Head" starts to play. The baby girl smiles and makes cheerful cries. If this moment of thriving and learning is one of many more to come, she will shine like a star throughout her life.

At the Kenwood Convent, Handel's "Water Music" is playing. An enthusiastic audience of retired Sisters of the Sacred Heart encircles the activities aide. The elders in wheelchairs or with walkers beside them stretch their arms vigorously like timeless wave riders on a glorious sea.

These are two scenarios of opposite places in life. Yet they show how wonderful beginnings and lonely endings may share the spontaneous discoveries that evoke joy awakened by attentive caregiving.

For a dozen years I have been helping caregivers develop programs using song and traditions in activities for older people. A decade before that, I'd begun recording lullabies in New York City to broaden the appeal of poetry and creative communication for an audience of all ages.

I am a Lullabologist…

When Ben Farnsworth produced a piece for WNBC television on the Lullaby Project, he reported: "Julia Lebentritt calls herself a **'Lullabologist.'** She has assembled a 60-minute tape of sleepytime around the city — music that has closed the eyes of generations." So it was the journalist who gave me the name that crystallized my calling. I **am** a lullabologist, which means that I study the role of lullabies and musical communications in the transitional passages of a person's life.

People often think of lullabies only as a way to put their children to sleep. But in speaking with parents and caregivers, I realized they also want permission to relax and connect with their loved ones. As important as putting the baby to sleep is the communication it encourages. I witnessed not only a repertory of stories, songs and images, but also gestures, routines and human interaction. I collected not just music, but a multitude of intimate experiences as adults and children learned from and healed each other.

Gradually I came to the discovery that my life work in world lullabies strikes notes for every generation. *As Long as You Sing, I'll Dance* is devoted to pushing the darkness back, offering caregiving skills that I call reciprocal caregiving. In this book I explain how all those responsible for the well-being of others can share the legacy of joyful and spontaneous caregiving.

My lullaby work has flowed into caregiving for the elderly who are often forgotten and end their lives in solitude. Newborn helplessness exists beside hope and growth. Old age helplessness can be reduced to a running down to a final stop. This need not be. We must value the dignity of vibrant relationships between caregivers and the elderly and the dying.

In this time of searches for alternative energy and sustainable systems, I propose that caregivers take this course in an alternative type of caregiving powered by feelings and relationships. I promise a dynamic experience for caregivers who are willing to apply discovered and recovered skills.

My approach, affirmed by compassionate voices as well as professional caregivers, is a "new" way because of my application of the traditions of lullaby singing. What I am adding is that this is a tradition for all ages. While I have learned a great deal about the manifestations of Alzheimer's disease and other debilitating illnesses and about interventions for managing goals, the wellspring of my method is deep human respect and love for the souls of others.

A newborn baby's performances evoke spontaneous communications that lead to mutual exchanges and bonding. The benefits of this time of love, thriving and open nurturing promote well-being and safekeeping. The same spontaneity of movement and communications works with infant, child, adult and elder. Caregivers can improve the quality of life and promote the independence of those whom they care for.

Older people with or without Alzheimer's disease and other dementias want to communicate with us even though they often can no longer do so directly. As their caregivers we must do the greater part in securing an understanding of their needs, their feelings and communications.

What I have found is staff members (whether or not responsible for activities) need both education about dementia and also help finding simple ways to connect and care. In my trainings and tools I help caregivers take the steps to care directly with loving kindness for others. Understanding the simplicity with which men and women who are memory impaired can look at things gives us a better understanding of how to approach sensitive and humane caregiving.

My vision for writing this creative arts activities guide is to help people discover the purpose behind communications while caregiving. All the activities are set within positive therapeutic fields of life-recall, storytelling, deep spontaneous imagery, guided imagery, expressive arts and complementary therapies. All the activities identify modes of pleasure that are available to you as a caring caregiver.

I hope this book reveals the wonderful ways that your own body and breath can use rhythm in its every guise to provide care and heal others and yourself. Every rainbow I have the chance to catch repeats the covenant of my mother's loving care. I offer these many ways of caregiving in the spirit of the Native American cradleboard that is empowered with turquoise appealing to the core and care of an individual.

While I am writing to champion a growing number of people who are underestimated, underserved, sometimes literally left to die, this book is also for the caregivers themselves whose spontaneous powers may have been zapped at an early age by traumatic events in basic human relationships. People need to be getting care especially when they are giving care. Caring for yourself is at the heart of my book of activities for caregivers.

Julia Soto Lebentritt

The 24/7 Caregiver's Lullaby

While close I hold thee in mine arms,
And sing my lullaby,
I think – what could become of thee
If I should chance to die?

From
*Lullabies of many lands collected
and rendered into English verse*
Alma Strettell, editor
Publisher George Allen, London, 1896

PART ONE

Following the Thread of Our Mothers' Joyful Caregiving

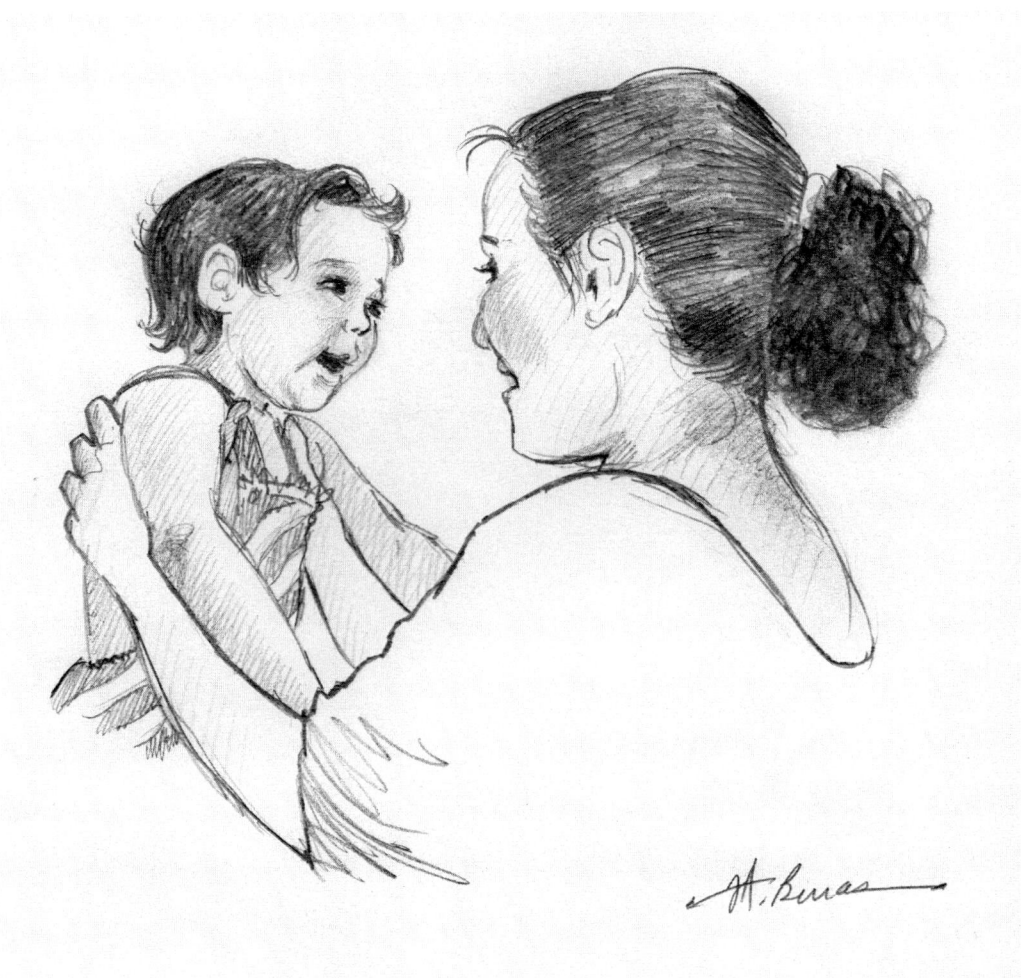

TAMMY & MELODY
*When people see children, even if not their own,
their instinct is to coo, smile and chat.*

ONE
When you're a caregiver, you're passing on the legacy of caregiving

It seems we could never forget these caregiving ways…

We can follow the thread of continuity in our life experiences of getting care and giving care. The thread of attachment is in healthy supportive communications found in ancient and universal traditions. Attachment begins with something that connects us.

Mothers and fathers accomplish these tireless connections day and night through magical caregiving. Some people connect to their children and families by cooking and baking favorite cherry pies, using old family and new cookbook recipes. Others travel, ferrying their charges to games, schools, dance lessons, parties, shops and back home again. Making wishes come true through the ages, caregivers bond. Their work proves positive when the people they cared for return the caring they received to the next generations. That is the legacy of joyful caregiving.

My mother used thread to sew us together with white lace christening dresses, graduation gowns, subtle silky underwear and flowered flannel nighties. Her movements were physical and emotional. She usually sewed in silence meditating, I fancy, on our happiness and our desires.

In 2003, in upstate New York, I rediscovered the skills of sewing that my mother taught me while teaching the residents of the Troy YWCA. Using all sorts of old sewing machines we stitched together in a project called "Sewing for Survival."

A local seamstress was our visiting teacher. Eleni immigrated from Greece, married and helped raise her family by sewing for Cluett & Peabody (makers of Arrow shirts) in the 1970s. Eleni bossed the YWCA women. In a shrill voice she shouted – "Put your foot *down* on the pedal!"

The women uneasy and fearful could not control the sewing machines. They were unaware of their ability to coordinate their bodies in order to sew for survival. Their modern shoes were awkward – clumsy styles too wide on the foot pedals that were designed for daintier footwear. They could not feel the pedal or contact it properly.

Like Eleni, my mother was an old–fashioned woman born in the first half of the 20th century. She passed on empowering skills that increase self-esteem, individuality and economic independence. The ability to survive includes providing shelter for the body by way of clothing as well as home, food, healthcare and loving caring relationships.

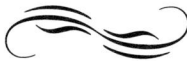

> Wolf learns to be a wolf through its mother.
> Bear learns to be a bear through its mother.
> Bird learns to be a bird through its mother.

Part of how mothers acculturate their children is bonding through musical language. Bonding through the use of simple rhythmic movements and vibrational verbalizations nurtures and grounds both the caregiver and the caregetter. Bonding cannot be done through materialism but only through relationship.

The earliest attachment, the placenta, surrounds the embryo, linking the umbilical cord to the womb of the mother. In fact, usually it takes universally nine months of womb life to produce a human life. When we are born we continue not as an afterthought or backup woman or man but as the inheritor of an individual form of life made by our mother's body's ability to attach, feed, nourish and pump out wastes during our embryonic beginnings. We look for what happened there in that embryonic sea for the meaning of our lives.

> Old navel,
> is this the spot
> where she last touched me?
> Oldest, first to die,
> was your connection me or her,
> or both of us?
> We both lost something then to begin with.
> Something between us died
> so she could walk separately and I could live outside.
> I nearly died alone many times.
> I built a cherry river branch for another's short life.
> Is this the face of Buddha once inside us,
> this doorknob-less grave of her and a nine-month-old child?
> And why do I go back to her
> as if the blood still rushed between us?
> There are others who look more like me.
> We could assume the same fantastic history
> looking for the explanation of our lives.

We experience a healthy sense of security and belonging in our mother's womb because we hear our own heartbeat echoed by our mother's heartbeat for nine months. The first placental palace is full of the natural rhythms of our mother's daily life, including her breathing, her burps, her laughter, her sobbing, her subtle sounds and her singing. Moved, rocked in this usually calm sea, our placental paradise provides a humming and singing entity full of safety. When we are born, this safe place and the first heartbeat disappear. We often go through life trying to find this rhythmic haven of the first heartbeat.

The first step upon being born is experiencing duality. We must cry and labor for milk and bread from birth on. Becoming separate independent human beings outside our mother now means we must learn to identify her and other separate beings by re-enacting or creating healthy attachments over and over, and over again.

The role of lullaby-songs and stories and singing to children in the world today is the same as ever. Lullabies function to create a safe attachment so that all that goes with the lullaby – the process, the ritual, the song, the singing voice – is internalized and the baby can let go, fall asleep, be alone without the mother (her voice, body, lap, breasts) near. The baby can then feel the certainty and the predictability that the day and the lullabies will always come back.

It seems we could never forget these caregiving ways and traditions that we inherit. Yet on street corners, at the mall and in other public places, we often hear the unanswered cries of a restless child, isolated and angry in a stroller beside adult caregivers who are often their clueless parents. Music cannot live without a dance. Is joyful caregiving no longer popular because the mothers, the fathers, we all are overworked? Where are the hushing, humming, chanting, playful ways of intervening and negotiating peace? The slow loss of the capacity to practice joyful caregiving is ultimately a loss of not only our own need for soothing and being soothed, but also our passion for being kept safe and calm. This oral tradition is passed from generation to generation. When a child who was sung to sleep in a nightly bedtime ritual becomes a mother and shifts to recorded music or no bedtime routine at all, she will feel less connected to her child and herself. Both parent and child will not know how to put their bodies into their voices – and their voices into their bodies. What is passed on from grandparent to parent to grandchild has changed dramatically in the past century.

Mary Catherine Bateson continues her mother Margaret Mead's insightful commentaries in *Peripheral Visions*: "The deepest changes may take generations with old attitudes concealed beneath efforts to adapt. My mother once commented that when a woman who was herself breastfed shifts to bottle feeding, she still holds her infant as she was held, as if nourishment were coming from her body; but when her daughter bottle-feeds, the echo is lost."

The failure to pass on this primary caregiving tradition leads to conflict, insecure families and a need for intervention therapies not only in childcare but also in adult and elder care. Too often, rushed caregivers at home and professional caregivers in retirement communities, nursing homes and hospitals fail to respond in intuitive ways to those in their care. If practices that enable people to make attachments and express elemental emotions are not carried on, then we may lose our memories of what it is to be human and our ability to be human.

An elder pleads for gentle caregiving

In 1996, I began working with senior citizens and persons with dementia and Alzheimer's, first as a case manager and counselor and then as an activities program director at a residential facility in Albany, New York. The director of nursing asked me to create a special care program for our most needy residents with memory deficiencies.

The Alzheimer's Association's Activity-Based Alzheimer's Care (ABAC) interactive training gave me an incredible perspective on ways to improve therapeutic care for the elderly. The ABAC manual says activities are the foundation of care, everyone interacts, and everyone is on the team. There are real challenges to implementing the innovative ABAC approach, and that's where reciprocal caregiving comes into play.

Before the special care programming, the residents with advancing dementias often sat in hallways sleeping or staring at one another. Their dignity as individuals went unrecognized. Without compassion and a therapeutic approach, few caregivers could know they were reachable, needed reaching and still had sharable human stories and cherished identities as our elders in the community.

I remember Betty, an 88-year-old retired teacher, pulling me aside one day to report an incident. She shook her fists and whispered, "She was rough lifting my legs onto the bed." Betty practically spat the words in disgust. "They need to treat us like *babies*!" She gestured with both arms cradling herself slowly rocking. "We cannot do everything for ourselves. They need to treat us gently. Talk with us and work slowly." Comparing herself to a baby needing tender love and care instead of a sick elderly patient needing lots of help, Betty kindled my own memories of the mutual enjoyment of caring for children. In addition, she catalyzed my discovery of using the intimate communications and rhythmic movements of lullaby traditions in activities.

My approach to the care of people with dementia or Alzheimer's builds on attachment-focused research begun more than 50 years ago by John Bowlby and Mary Ainsworth and the work of Barry Reisberg, a New York psychiatrist who coined the term "retrogenesis" to describe the way the mind's deterioration reflects its development; the first faculties to develop are the last to go. So it is that people with memory loss respond to stimulations that call forth their former routines, jobs, home life, hobbies and often deceased loved ones. So it is that people with dementia can often sing, read, play an instrument, reminisce, tell stories and dance when they have difficulty maintaining a conversation. Even when they do not remember the people or places from day to day, people with dementia remember the feelings associated with places and people. Objects like fishing rods, familiar tools, towels to be folded and pictures of loved ones trigger and restore connections with remembered selves. Positive repetitive experiences like replaying a song and asking for the same story over and over again allow those with dementia to act in their environment. Traditional lullaby routines build on these skills and habits with the goal of improving quality of life and independence by using strengths.

> **Spreading John Zeisel's good news**
>
> "The good news is that a great deal is going on in there even as our brains get plaques, tangles, cavities, folds and fissures. Our brains contain hard-wired, universal, preexisting images and abilities – sometimes called instincts or natural feelings. These immediately accessible abilities that help all of us to communicate in a split second with each other are equally useful in enabling people living with Alzheimer's to communicate with us and we with them."
>
> "Because preexisting hard-wired characteristics, memories, and skills are acquired even before birth, the theory of "retrogenesis" would lead us to infer that these may never be lost in the brain and mind of a person living with Alzheimer's. They are always present, accessible to the person, and are therefore the building blocks for successful communication and continuing relationships."
>
> From *I'm Still Here: A breakthrough approach to understanding someone with Alzheimer's* by John Zeisel

My special approach to care and management, reciprocal caregiving, evokes caregivers' past experiences as children and/or caregivers of children to transfer a way of understanding and approaching caregiving. All the activities in this book appeal to the hard-wired parts of the brain that we do not forget via musical communications; visual images and visualizations; sense of home and safety; nature; facial expressions; touch; rhythmic movements, singing and drumming; and just plain helping each other.

This creative approach can be as playful and loving as interactions between parents and their young children. A 90-year-old may exhibit the same symptoms as a six-month-old – disorientation about person, place and time; failure to recognize familiar caregivers; physical needs; incontinence; agitated behavior; screaming; and erratic sleep patterns. The aged person is just as lovable as the child.

"Those ending their lives in the helplessness of old age deserve the same care and attention as those beginning their lives in the helplessness of infancy," Dr. Paul E. Ruskin reports in *Journal of the American Medical Association*. But it is not easy. He contends that the reason it is much more difficult is because "the infant represents new life, hope, and utmost potential; the demented senior citizen, on the other hand, represents the end of life, with little potential for growth."

Don't *baby* me! Just take care of me with kindness

In a 2008 *New York Times* story headlined, "In 'Sweetie' and 'Dear,' a Hurt for the Elderly," John Leland writes: "Professionals call it elderspeak, the sweetly belittling form of address that has always rankled older people."

The term "elderspeak" derives from what has been alternately approved and disapproved of by various child development professionals: namely baby talk, motherese, parentese, mommy talk, caretaker speech, infant directed talk (IDT) and child-directed talk (CDT).

Researchers in the field of gerontology have documented that elderspeak can diminish older people's confidence in their abilities. "Despite such research," Leland warns us, "the worst offenders are often health care workers." However, at least one person quoted in his article gives an opposite opinion, "If someone calls us sweetie or honey, it's not diminishing us; it's just their way to connect, in a positive way." In the New Old Age Blog, "Elders on Elderspeak," Leland writes, "The question of elderspeak and the vehemence of disagreement over it gets at one of the vexing issues of aging: the lack of a language on which people of different walks agree. Some like the words 'dear,' 'sweetie,' 'senior,' 'elderly,' 'aged' and 'old' – or at least consider them neutral. To others, they are a source of dissonance."

I am not advocating that caregivers revert to baby talk when communicating with seniors any more than Betty was asking for baby talk when she showed me – wrapping her arms lovingly around herself and rocking gently – how she wanted her caregivers to treat her and others in their care. In fact, her reference to "rough lifting" generated a report of possible abuse to the director. Clearly, her request to be treated gently, slowly and with kind words indicated that some staff members might be mechanically putting the dependent elders to bed with hasty, risky moves rather than a caring, therapeutic respectful touch. Caring communications can become a way to help us relate more kindly and deeply to others.

Should language be controlled or user-friendly? At an assisted-living retirement community in Vermont where I worked, the director suddenly decided without consulting staff or residents that the residents should be addressed always and only by titles and their last names. When the staff polled the residents, they unanimously rejected being called Mr. or Mrs. or Miss or Doctor and supported the current usage of first names. These residents did not want to revert to a formal relationship code in their new home in a continuing-care retirement community.

We all speak the same language as caregivers because caregiving is holistic. One of Mother Teresa's favorite sayings describes this approach: "Show kindness through your face, your eyes, your smile and through the warmth of your greetings. You must bear a cheerful smile. Don't only give your care, but give your heart as well."

So the language of caregiving (body language as well) is organic and natural, sometimes urgent and critical, not insulting or derogatory as long as the attitude behind our communications is positive and supportive. In my opinion, "elderspeak" becomes a way of disconnecting from a relationship when the form and tone of a greeting express a negative or ambivalent estimation of someone's value. In other words don't *baby* me with elderspeak. Just take care of me with kindness.

May we all become more spontaneous, enjoy the small things in life, become less product-oriented, more process-oriented, and release ourselves from withdrawn patterns of relationship.

But use caution. Do not take your spontaneity lightly. Nor is it another burden or additional responsibility. The intent is to help you relate, tuning into inner harmony first then finding the tune (as well as what name someone wants to be called) together.

My goal in this book is to share the gift of being alive. This presents a way for caregivers to enter the world of someone who is ill or suffering with cognitive loss modeled on the ways that parent caregivers enter the world of their children.

Not everyone knows how to inspire and recognize the communications that I call first song-signs of life – a light in the eyes, a tap of the toes, a catcall meow. An attentive caregiver can pick up on a feeling or a look that others miss. Slow the pace for a moment and grab a hand and obtain an understanding of people beyond their disability. Instill hope. Provide sustaining communications and mind-body-spirit healing.

> "La la, lu lu, do do, bye bye – these sounds take us back. Before birth the powerful drumbeat of the mother's heart promises a secure rhythm."
>
> "New York Lullabies" CD Track 7 "Mother's Heartbeat"

TWO
When you are a spontaneous caregiver, you are in a happily developing relationship

I am offering these creative arts activities as a therapy for those who are traumatized by illness, isolation and depression and who need relationships, safety and stability as much as the completely dependent children who first inspire lullaby singing.

> ### The caregiver's challenge
>
> Carol Bowlby Sifton describes the challenge in *Navigating the Alzheimer's Journey: A Compass for Caregiving* this way: "Caregivers face the challenge of creatively bypassing the disease-induced losses in ways of maintaining conventional connectedness – to find ways without words – to reveal and experience relationships on other planes."

Relationships can be identified as movement between two people. Moving too fast and moving too slow in the relationship process can put our communications out of sync. In a sense we all are, or often feel we are, out of sync, alone and separate from each other. Our daily work schedules put us out of sync with our own bodies' natural rhythms and needs. The caregiver has to move with those at risk, start where they are, and meet them there before they can move forward together. A sharing experience is brought about by each partner adapting to the other's spontaneous interests and activities.

Here are two examples of spontaneous caregiving relationships:

1. Edward

An activities assistant comes back from a music and movement session. She tells another staff member: "Edward knew all the words to the first song on the CD. I read the words to him checking them line by line. He *knew* all the words!" The elderly gentleman in her care is in early stages of cognitive loss. Edward may not understand the meanings of the words, but he can remember the feeling of accomplishment and independence of hearing and singing the familiar song. This feeling becomes associated with the place and time of music and movement sessions, and it begins to feel like home whenever we play this particular song.

2. Sylvia

In another setting, song sheets cover the table where Sylvia sits in her pillowed wheelchair. Suddenly Sylvia starts engaging with the song sheets, shuffling and sorting them. Staring at one page, holding it up, she acts like she is reading the words aloud. She recites: "Twinkle, star. Are you are? In the night lighting tonight."

Sylvia's voice is ethereal as if coming from a million miles away. Her aged face glows. She recognizes a familiar routine. Actually, this usually reclusive elder is praying the words. Caregivers can stimulate the recall of words and skills such as reading, writing, singing, reciting familiar rhymes and prayers or playing an instrument.

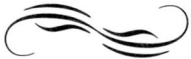

In both of these responses, the people in our care acted spontaneously. We did not plan ahead that Edward would remember the words and sing along or that Sylvia would interact with the scattered song sheets instead of the music that the caregiver was playing. Both responses began with their perceptions and spontaneous attention.

As caregivers, we attended sensitively to their interests and tendencies. We did not try to change their responses. This is the essence of spontaneous care communications. In the Maria Montessori method, young children learn best when they direct their own learning with teachers providing the tools that engage all their senses. "We discovered that education is not something the teacher does," Montessori wrote, "but a natural process that develops spontaneously in the human being."

People with memory deficiencies also respond when they can "learn" through their own hands and muscle memory as well as their eyes and brains. Elders with dementia and disabilities are hearing, feeling human beings in need of enlightened humane care. Of course, they are learning – learning to live with cognitive loss and other losses, learning how to deal with what is eventually a terminal illness. I promise they will give back more happiness and satisfaction than ever imagined when cared for with love and care.

Spontaneity is not learned

We are born with dynamic capabilities. We are the artist's brush poised to dip our voices and bodies into colors and media like water colors, oils, and pastels. We can vibrate, whirl, become multiple passions and weave endless threads in our lifetime and beyond time as we know it by the clocks. Often unhealthy practices move into our bodies, tiring us, dulling our fresh skills, making us sick, old, numb, unhappy, unloved and unlovable. Blocked by our addictions we cannot make room in our bodies for enriching traditions, repertories and free creative solutions especially when the repertories and traditions are not passed along. When secrets are kept – when true feelings are repressed for generations – we become strangers who think we know everything about others while we do not begin to know ourselves.

Advocacy for compassionate care of people with cognitive impairments like Alzheimer's, including new ways to connect to the person not the disease, is growing. In his recent book, *I'm Still Here,* John Zeisel, an innovator in non-pharmacological approaches to treatment of Alzheimer's affirms my belief in using the old ways, instincts, natural feelings and the creative arts to enable people living with Alzheimer's to communicate with us and we with them.

As Long as You Sing, I'll Dance redefines the field of caregiving. Care partners need to rediscover their relational well-being in order to care for themselves and others using the old ways, instincts and natural feelings. The innate ability to be sensitive to emotional expressions and responsive to other people's needs is in need of rescue and revitalization.

We who are the partners are living on a traumatized planet in the 21st century. We are slowly realizing the effects of an unstable economy and global greenhouse disasters. Too often we are also coming from dysfunctional families and emotionally deprived relationships. *As Long as You Sing, I'll Dance* can help all those who are caring caregivers care for themselves as well.

This book will help you apply creative parenting methods and traditions that are calming and soothing to ill people who often exhibit agitated, anxious and disturbing behaviors that are considered unmanageable and challenging. It is for those who are dependent and SUPPORTS those who want to help them.

Spontaneous & Reciprocal Care Essentials

Care is about what comes naturally to a person; it is not about what comes from constraint or external stimulus.

Care is about according dependent people heart-to-heart care; it is not about discord or suppression.

Care is about responding in actions and words with joyful communications; it is not about withholding.

Care is about placing trust in your ability to agree with transitions; it is not about your inflexible idea of youth, yourself and aging.

Care is about being interested and present; it is not about wishing you were somewhere else.

Care is about the breath you take with gratitude; it is not about the life you take for granted.

Care is about the care you grant with love; it is not about keeping secrets about whom and what you love.

The underlying principles of spontaneous care communications are:
- Empowerment of individuals (who are trained professionals and untrained community members alike)
- The caregiving potential of people of all ages for people of all ages
- Commonality of our communication abilities
- Human responsibility and inborn abilities to interact in situations
- Relationships as movements between two or more people.

THREE
Caring is about something much larger than caregiving

By putting care in the context of parenting, I hope to get people to care more about what they are doing.

"To care" has a constellation of interrelated meanings. "Care" as defined under "feelings" in Roget's Thesaurus means "to emotionally respond":

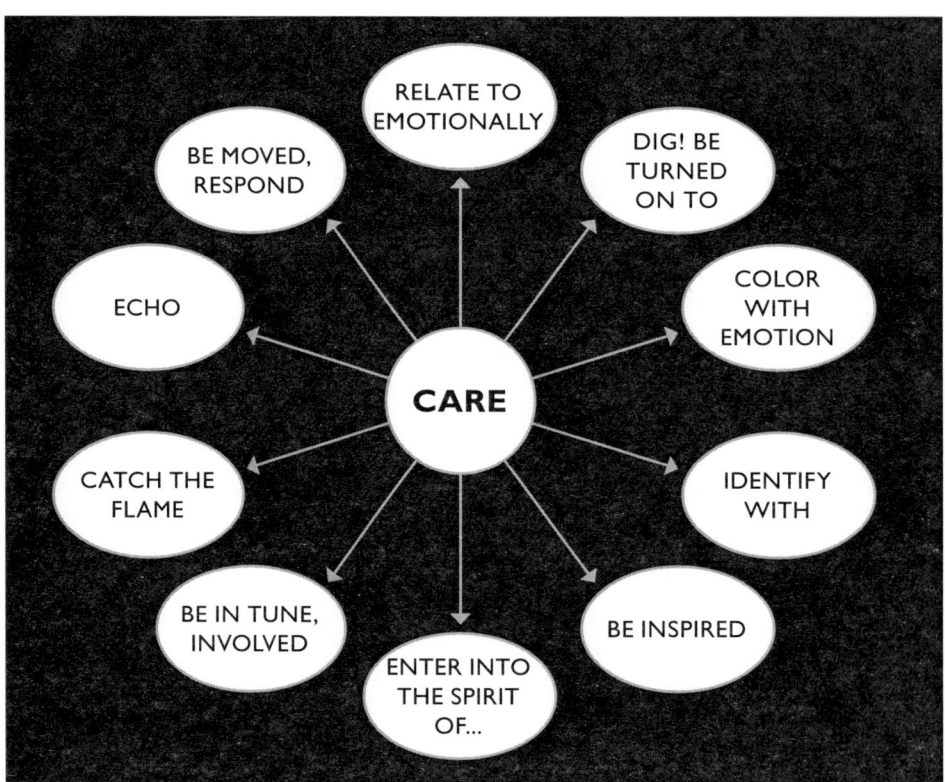

Almost all the words in this chart are emotional words for "care." This activities guidebook offers innovative approaches to caring. This kind of care originates from spontaneity in the natural communications and bonding between children and parents.

Reciprocal care summons our own and others' feelings. The legacy of lullaby traditions worldwide is never just music. It is movement, dance and speech, and so it is a form of spontaneous musical care in which each person is involved not just as a listener but as a performer. It allows us to tap into emotional and intuitive powers that are sensory, subjective, interpretive and sincere. Lullabies provide interactive ways of keeping parents in the present of their own parenting experience and remembering their own childhood.

Like trains on rails, we attempt to run our lives on schedules. Caregivers need schedules and routines and plans. They also need to access, assess and apply compassion and creative talents. To be more whole-brained in our caregiving requires giving equal weight to the spontaneous activities, arts, imagination and synthesis. Left brain functions are routine, and planned. Right brain functions are creative, sensitive and compassionate. Schools tend to focus on logical thinking, analysis and accuracy, which connect to left brain.

Illustration: The Problem

Discuss left-brain versus right-brain thinking in caregiving using "The Problem" of Caroline not wanting to go into the dining room to eat:

Just before supper, Caroline insists she wants to go to her room. As the activities aide pushes Caroline in her wheelchair past the dining room, the nursing assistant calls out to her: "Where are you taking her? She can't go to her room. It's suppertime!"

What's wrong here?

Discussion of The Problem

The nursing assistant is "going by the book." Task-and schedule-oriented, she confronts both Caroline and the aide, angering them by not addressing either of them by name. The tone of voice, "calling out," is disruptive to everyone in the dining room who is beginning to relax and enjoy dinner. There is no recognition, consideration or negotiation offered by the nursing assistant regarding the reasons why Caroline wants and/or needs to go to her room.

There is no emotional team support in the nursing staff member's approach to the activities staff member. Also, there is a lack of understanding and education regarding Caroline's cognitive loss.

> ### The return to the first language
>
> "Nonverbal communication – first language, the unspoken language of the body again becomes the most important language," Carol Bowlby Sifton wrote extensively about communicating with someone with dementia in *Navigating the Alzheimer's Journey*. "For persons with dementia, the return to the first language is difficult because of our lifelong, adult focus on verbal communications."

My special approach to care and management evokes caregivers' past experiences as children and/or caregivers of children to transfer a way of understanding and approaching care. If your personal communication style has always included much touch and gesture, this may be easier. The activities offer practices that activate the unspoken language of the body, touch, facial expressions, voice tone, body posture and gestures.

You may believe that caregivers who act spontaneously don't know their boundaries, but I have seen that spontaneous communication opens up blocked and stagnant confining states of mind and body. Acting and communicating spontaneously may feel very scary, even as if you are acting without thinking. But I've seen – like magic of childhood – genies emerge to move energies in our lives.

On the other hand one administrator in a retirement community where people needing all levels of care were separated into skilled, assisted and independent units with locked doors was very outspoken about keeping the special care dementia people away from others. "Those people are spontaneous," she contended. "They don't know their borders, and they should not be allowed into community reunions."

I argued that residents would benefit from each other. Other administrators agreed with me and we brought all the residents together for special events. At one of them Marianne, a plucky elder who suffered cognitive loss and a hearing disability in her nineties, demanded her own paper and pencil when we passed out a word game. In the next five minutes, she made up just as many words as the best of them, all spelled and written correctly. To everyone's delight Marianne won a prize. The other elders exchanged glowing smiles.

When a person's behavior is described as "poor short term memory," it is viewed as a problem that requires a solution. When the same behavior is described as spontaneous, it may be viewed as a positive characteristic, not something to stop, control, fix or restrict.

Unrehearsed communications can warm and excite everyone, lighting eyes with the brightest love. That is because spontaneous communications like music affect everyone's brain waves or the "rhythms" of our brains, creating more brainpower that charges us in a present moment of unified community spirit.

When you learn to give yourself permission to be spontaneous, you will start to melt mountains and break through the barbed wire fences that separate us.

Illustrations of spontaneous communications

The day nurse forgets herself, and she dances into the middle of the Christmas sing-along shouting, "Joy to the World! That's my favorite song!"

She even grabs the microphone singing with all her heart "repeat the sounding joy…" Then as she exits, someone calls, "There goes Joy – our joy to the world." Her vibrant movements fill the halls and connect everyone to a vital passionate universal love of life, song and confidence.

Mimi, the playful secretary, takes a break from her desk and saunters into the waiting room. She shakes a finger at a restless elder who is waiting in line for the dentist while she sings "You better watch out, you better not cry." Laughter ripples the crowd and enhances the social skills we need to make friends and handle problems.

FOUR
Care about what they care about

Sometimes we say and do things that have no relationship to the people we are with. We may be talking and moving out of sync with each other even when we are intimates lying in the same bed together, partners in business sitting across the table from each other or providers performing services for others – pitching a million dollar deal or spoon-feeding a dependent child or adult.

Take Wilma's window, for example: Wilma points to the window. "This is my window up to where the blue flower is." She shows me the invisible line that is drawn down the middle of the room that she shares with a roommate in the nursing home.

"All the nurses care about is the curtains!" Wilma says she fights with the nurses every night. "They don't care about the window." Wilma grumbles on to herself about the losing battle she has since she moved into the skilled care wing and went on hospice care.

Wilma loves looking out the wide window at the western sky. She sees men flying home from Albany to Schenectady at five o'clock. We look but we cannot see the planes they fly in.

There's a tall pine tree and other trees that Wilma and her roommate talk about. "Too bad they close the curtain," I commiserate. "Maybe you could wake up and see the moon in the sky there."

This triggers beautiful memories for both women. When they lived in the assisted living unit, they managed to go outside to the courtyard. Despite the staff's protests, they waited for the full moon to rise over the pine tree. The nurses were afraid they would get pneumonia but they demanded to watch the sky until the moon rose over the pine trees.

In this all too common example, Wilma says, "All the nurses care about is the curtains!" The nurses do not care about the window that Wilma cares about because she wants to look out the window at the changing twilight in the sky.

The nurses may be forced to care about clinical regulations and compliance issues. The curtains must be closed on the window because of privacy, safety or other issues. In this case, in order to care about what Wilma cares about it may be possible and necessary to bring this problem up at a Care Plan meeting and write an order for the curtains to be left open at sunset so Wilma does not exhibit angry combative behaviors that may lead to depression and social withdrawal. With caring communications, we can care about what someone else cares about even in a clinically regulated setting.

Too often we are so intent on our own paths and the rules that we mistake our actions as caregivers as caregiving when the caregetter wants a much different caring activity.

Can you adjust your schedule spontaneously when a person you care for asks you to sit down and talk with him or her a while? Can you sit and talk and listen?

It is often the personal caregivers, the nurse assistants or home health aides who are the people in whom hospice patients want to confide their true feelings about dying. Can we allow ourselves and others to care about what the caregetter cares about?

Going along with this more humane caregiving approach, can we care about what they would care about if they could? For example, if the patient's feet are frozen in advanced stages of dementia – if she's no longer able to perform her own activities of daily living and obviously needs to be adjusted in her bed or chair before a meal is served – wouldn't she, wouldn't you care about getting your toes free of covers and not smashed against the foot of the bed?

Dependent adults require the same thoughtful care as dependent babies who cannot walk or turn themselves in cribs. It takes only a few moments to adjust our activities and assess the actual situation and environment in which we are performing. When you enter the caregetter's room as a caregiver, pause and try to see what she sees, feels, says or doesn't say. To be a thoughtful caregiver doesn't mean to be lost in thoughts out there in the stratosphere but to be engaging in caring responsibly. Think about what they care about while you care. Active listening and validation of others' situations puts us in gear for spontaneous and reciprocal caregiving.

FIVE
Your spontaneous powers

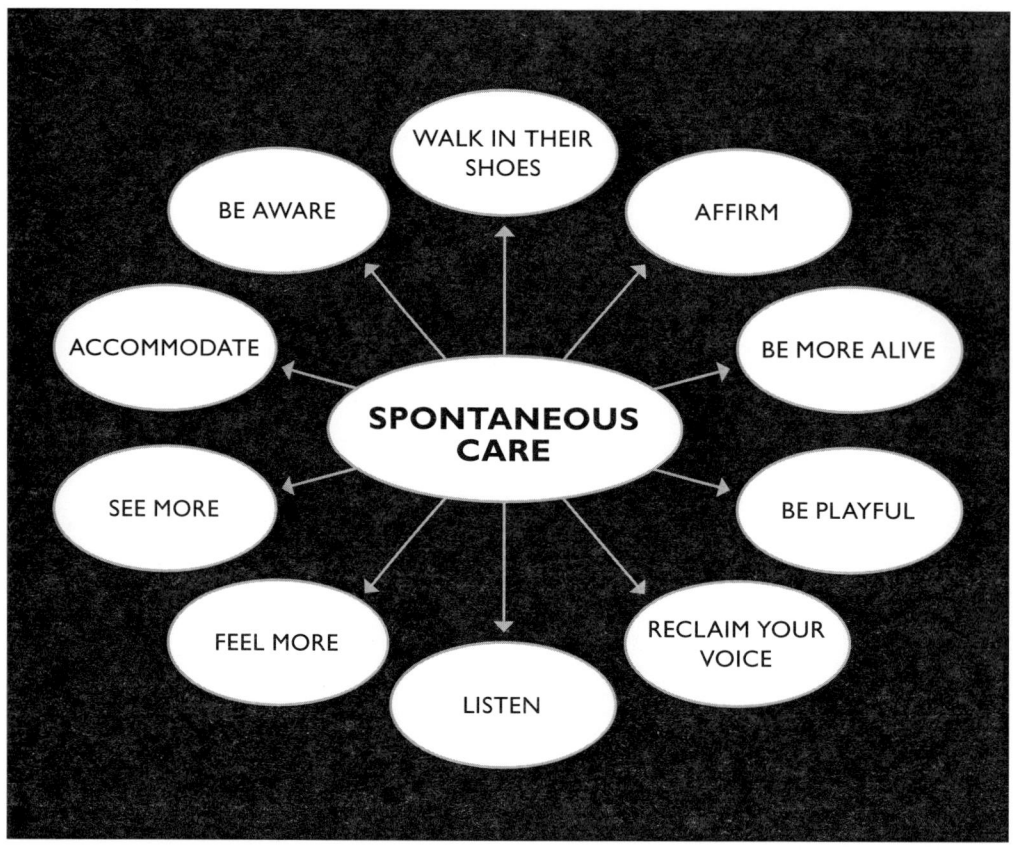

Listen

Listen to the way those in your care speak.

Interrupting and calling for them to stay on the subject and be correct does not work.

Listen for what they are saying, doing and/or not saying or doing. Often they are not using logical structures, or they may not be in the same time zone as you are.

Listen for emotional messages, indirect imagery and poetic language that convey the need behind otherwise confusing statements.

Examples: "I think I have a lily going to sleep."

"I hear the holly bush crying."

"Where's your duck?" (meaning your dog who usually visits with you)

Listen for echoes, repetitions.

Echo and repeat what you hear others say.

Redirect negative feelings to positive memories, places and/or people.

When Mary was able to speak long-distance with her mother on the phone on Mother's Day, she was pretty sure her mother recognized her voice although her mom then seemed to think Mary was *her* mother, and she was looking forward to her mother (not Mary) coming over to visit. Mary loved that her mother connected with her personal thoughts of her mother (long-dead) through her on Mother's Day.

When the nurse held the phone to her mother's ear, Mary savored her mother's "coos" and treasures this moment when they connected. She felt certain that she was recognized by her mother even though the recognition shifted to times long ago.

Connecting our elders to nurturing memories of earlier times supports and enriches communications. Instead of demanding that they keep track of the daily census, and doggedly pointing to all the family and friends long dead while announcing "I am your daughter now!" we can take delight in dementia's whimsical lights breaking through the clouds.

Feel more

> You are in the caregetter's play/field/dream, not vice versa.
> Feel for their comfort. Notice how the environment affects them.
> Is it too noisy, cold, warm *or* boring?
> Name things in their environment like colors, smells and other people.

See more

> Look for a light in the eyes, small gestures and subtle changes.
> Give direct attention, eye to eye, face to face and one to one.
> Assist elders so they can have direct contact with others.
> Position wheelchair people face to face near each other so they can reach for each other's hands and have conversations, however minimal.

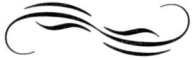

The wife of a nursing home patient speaks with conflicted feelings about visiting him. Something positive does happen for her however during her daily afternoon visits because she remembers with bubbling laughter – "I love to see these people light up. It takes me a half-hour just to get down the hall to his room."

Often he is reclining in a geri-chair – his eyes closed deeply lethargic – now and then rousing with a deep snore. She greets him several times. He opens his eyes briefly but remains non-verbal. His wife admits she becomes tearful and appreciative of any support.

An hour passes with very little change. His wife kisses his forehead and lips – strokes his cheeks saying "I love you honey" with intimate caring.

His eyes open slits then close, a slight beginning of a soft smile comes and goes. Then he falls back into his lethargic state both hands making fists. Clouds passing – sun breaking through intermittently. His wife now thinks with terror and fear about her own mother who also had Alzheimer's – "Oh, what a terrible, terrible disease!" Is there anything she can do for him? She strokes his hands slowly so they will relax and open and not freeze into fists.

She sings their wedding song a little – "Hopelessly Devoted to You." Next she goes to get him some thickened water. To her delight he begins to rouse after each sip. He mutters, and then finally begins to speak words in response.

"You like that?"

"I'll say…."

His eyes search like two lighthouse beams penetrating darkness. Blue eyes brimming, he drinks her in. It is as if he sees her for the first time. She teases him, "Are you okay?"

"OKAY?" he roars knowingly.

Be aware

More than seeing and listening, being aware means being completely present in the moment.

Getting to know my Spanish-speaking mother-in-law was difficult due to our language barrier. Then one day, we sat together with her three-year-old grandson on the concrete steps outside their Bronx home. In English and Spanish Mommy and I started to make up stories about the ants that were marching into sand hills as Michael laughed excitedly, joining in to name the ants and their antics. Our attention together on an ant hole brought to light a new understanding and relationship to cherish.

> *In learning to give reciprocal and spontaneous care:*
>
> ☐ Learn to care about yourself
>
> ☐ Recognize your own sensual pleasure
>
> ☐ Appreciate your knowledge
>
> ☐ Increase your capacity for giving and receiving quality care
>
> ☐ Affirm that your life, feelings and thoughts and surroundings are worth attention

Be more alive

Be a life-giving caregiver. Pass the flame of your keen perceptions with animated visibility.

To be more alive, use the thesaurus words for care: "to catch the flame."

To catch the flame brings to mind the Olympic flame carried by runners. In 2004, the first global torch relay was undertaken in a journey that lasted 78 days.

The power of catching and passing the flame in the Olympic torch relay is regularly enacted to facilitate communication in many expressive-arts group therapy warm-ups. The torch is passed as a koosch ball, balloon, peacock feather or bean bag in a circle or between partners. Words are added like the participants' names or other calls and responses.

This exercise serves to break through the disconnection among group members. Everyone responds to an immediate task like runners in a torch relay. As we catch the object we emotionally respond and relay the action to another member of the group passing on the need to respond to one another.

In these exercises we are always ready to respond (that is, care) because we may be relayed to again and again at any moment. We cannot throw to another person one time only and then sit down to watch the clock saying, "That's all you'll get from me!" Caring, caregiving, caregetting require a constant interactive readiness to respond.

Just as the light of the torch once kindled by the sun must be kept alive by the global runners, every day you are dancing the job of caregiving like a runner in a torch relay, keeping your eye on the need to keep the flame of your care burning by receiving and giving in the tradition of caregiving.

Make the purpose of your caregiving activities:

☐ Not to kill time but to make time live

☐ Not to keep yourself and other persons occupied but to keep yourself and others refreshed

☐ Not to offer an escape from life or mechanical maintenance of life but to provide a discovery of life

☐ Breathe life into each moment and create a dynamic interchange with the world

Walk in their shoes

The loss of physical and mental abilities that allow independence is associated with aging. This is a common denominator of human life. You can imagine what it will be like to not be able to see, walk, drive a car, go to work or communicate your needs or feelings.

Reverence for elders' hard-won wisdom engenders belief in the love of the smallest hopeful moment – a "meow," a comforting hand or a breath of fresh air.

When we walk in their shoes, we learn deep compassion for the essential nature of our journeys on this earth. This compassion connects us deeply to self-love, each other and healing.

When my colleague referred to people as "saddled with dementia," I explained my different perspective.

- These people can see your spirit more than other people.
- They are more right-brain, spontaneous in their intake and output.
- They are not trammeled with ego.
- They are childlike, imitative and playful.
- They are like mystics out there between cognitive worlds.

So I am asking you to be more like them and "walk in their shoes."

Trying to remember is very private and totally personal. Being uncertain about being able to remember a face, where you put your keys, when you were born, who you are, is for human beings a tragic loss of identity, purpose, meaning, faith and self-confidence — that light that we were born with.

For example: "I don't know if I can remember how to dance," the father of the groom confessed after the wedding.

He had looked very strict — angry when he was asked to dance with his son's new bride. All he betrayed was his aggressive absolutely certain "No!" — like a door shut in his son's face with no access evermore. It was later on the long drive home that he mentioned aloud as an after thought his uncertainty about trying to remember an everyday activity.

Of course he doesn't dance a lot, never did, but he did dance at his wedding and other weddings. When traditions cannot be followed due to some hidden disability, we often do not understand that there are cognitive and possibly other physical changes in our loved ones because they hide their private and frightened thoughts.

Like a search that freezes the computer — a lighthouse in thickest fog — an unborn child fading away, an aborted pregnancy — he did not dance with the bride because he didn't remember how to dance.

Accommodate

In talking with my Dominican neighbor, I learned about *canciones de cuna* – *songs of the cradle*.

Cuna is not only the cradle or crib. *Cuna* is the way the mother accommodates the baby. *Cuna* is the way the baby is held in arms, the crib, or any other place, thing or way provided for the baby's rest. Tammy told me that her mother used a drawer to cradle her. *Cuna* means origins, native land, home, family lineage, languages, food, songs, sounds – deep, deep culture specific to each person and place.

In caregiving, it is necessary to adjust to different needs and patterns, to negotiate and accommodate or make a "place" for another's wishes and rights to choose what they want, when they want it. It becomes a challenge to negotiate with a patient who often does not want to take the medicine now, or go to a community program now, but there are always options available to accommodate each other.

You can learn to communicate better when you accept that caregiving is a human exchange and subject to constant challenging behaviors to be negotiated and accommodated, despite your superior role as the caregiver of a dependent human being.

Make a cradle of each moment to hold your own and other's daily needs.

Be playful

This should be the most available power, yet it is often the hardest to find.

Why not just blow up a balloon, tie it off and toss it back and forth with a few people to see what a little fun can do for everyone?

Reclaim your voice

There is scientific evidence that very early musical responsiveness is an innate function in all human beings. Although radios, boom boxes and ipods can be easily placed in homes and institutions as a stimulus, caregivers' voices are always best.

> The sound of your own voice reassures that you are present and functioning.
>
> It reaffirms your personal identity.
>
> From Christine Knowles reflections on
> *As Long as You'll Sing, I'll Dance*

> Echo means to care. In Greek mythology, Echo, a mountain nymph, suffers a disastrous love affair that leaves her pining for the love she never knew until only her voice remains. Repeating the last words and sounds of others is so often a part of a mother's way of teaching her young child to communicate and learn the mother's language.
>
> To care, emotionally respond, we must listen, attend to others and repeat, echo them with our voice and body gestures. Think of standing alone on the shore of a lake or pond where you see no other sign of moving life except the water ripples, then calling, shouting across the water as if someone is there across on the other shore.
>
> There will be a delay after you let your call carry. Then vibrational energy returns your last words and sounds in a voice repeating over and over part of your own sound, voice and words.
>
> Eerie? No, this is the response of deeply connecting with our consciousness. Believe in the echo of your inner and outer self as you care for yourself and others.

Follow your own way and your own rhythms as you progress through reciproal caregiving training. You will quickly demonstrate that musical communications are not the property of the elite members of society or those with advanced educations. Each of you will be able to create songs and communicate with the people you care for and love in a personal and genuine way.

And affirm…

Do not hide your light under a basket.
Let it shine for all the world
And centuries to see.
—A variation on "St. Lucy's Prayer"

> The whole purpose of all this
> Is to trick people
> Into their own singing
> And song banks of memories.
> So when that happens
> Drop the book
> And sing along!

SIX
Free up your spontaneous powers quiz

At home we free up space in our computers, refrigerators, closets, cupboards, drawers, desks, jewel boxes, pocketbooks and cars. Otherwise, stuff builds up and blocks our activities.

In business we free up cash by making internal or external changes that will generate more revenue.

Why not free up our inborn ability to respond and communicate actively and originally?

Take your own vital signs using the spontaneous care communications song-signs of life quiz.

1) Do you know the words to any songs?
    A. Many.
    B. A few.
    C. None.

2) Do you read aloud to yourself?
    A. Often.
    B. Sometimes.
    C. Never.

3) Do you read aloud to others?
    A. Often.
    B. Sometimes.
    C. Never.

4) Do you hum, grunt, sigh, and moan?
   A.   Often.
   B.   Sometimes.
   C.   Never.

5) Do you talk and cry at the same time alone or in public?
   A.   Sometimes alone and in public.
   B.   Sometimes alone.
   C.   Sometimes in public.
   D.   Never.

6) Do you walk barefoot at home?
   A.   Often.
   B.   Sometimes.
   C.   Never.

7) Do you walk barefoot outside?
   A.   Often.
   B.   Sometimes.
   C.   Never.

8) Do you talk to animals?
   A.   Often.
   B.   Sometimes.
   C.   Never.

9) Do you talk to flowers, clouds or trees?
   A.   All of the above.
   B.   Some of the above.
   C.   None of the above.

10) How many times a day do you laugh out loud?
	A.	Many times.
	B.	Once or twice.
	C.	Never.

11) Can you still skip, jump or bounce a ball?
	A.	All of the above.
	B.	One or two of the above.
	C.	None of the above.

12) Do you create nicknames for your pets, plants or friends?
	A.	All of the above.
	B.	Some of the above.
	C.	None of the above.

13) Can you caw like a crow, neigh like a horse, meow like a cat, hiss like a snake or bah like a sheep?
	A.	All of the above.
	B.	Some of the above.
	C.	None of the above.

14) Do you mix your jackets and pants?
	A.	Often.
	B.	Sometimes.
	C.	Never.

15) Do you look for several possible solutions to a problem?
	A.	Often.
	B.	Sometimes.
	C.	Never.

16) How often do you tell your own stories?
    A. Often.
    B. Sometimes.
    C. Never.

17) How often do you listen to the stories of others?
    A. Often.
    B. Sometimes.
    C. Never.

18) How many nursery rhymes can you recite by heart?
    A. More than five.
    B. Three.
    C. None.

19) When you watch a fireworks display, do you cheer, jump, clap, talk or gesture to strangers in the crowd?
    A. Cheer, jump, clap most of the time as well as greet others.
    B. Cheer most of the time – never talk to strangers.
    C. Cheer, jump, clap only at the end and never talk to strangers.
    D. Clap only at the end.
    E. None of the above.

20) When you get a fortune cookie, what do you do?
    A. Always open it and read the fortune aloud.
    B. Sometimes open it and read the fortune aloud.
    C. Always open it, never read fortune aloud.
    D. Never open the fortune cookie – or eat it.

Rating system for the Free Up Your Spontaneous Powers Quiz:

Straight A's
indicates your song-signs of life are hale and hearty.

Any B's or C's or D's
indicate it would be good for your health to work toward an A score.

PART TWO
Rhythmic Movements and Spontaneous Songs

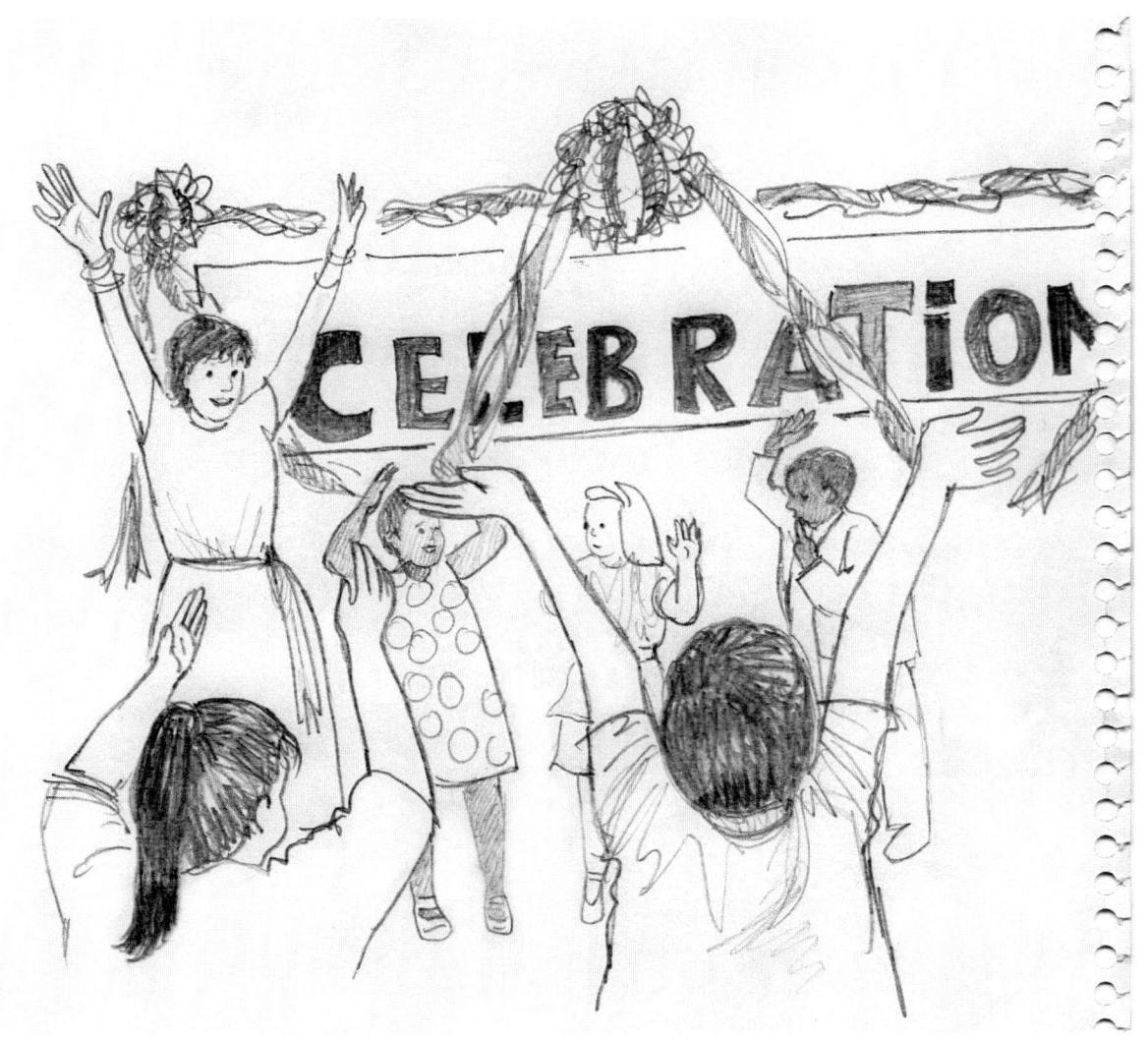

JULIA & KINDERGARTEN
The visiting artist uses songs to introduce characteristic body movements of dance and traditional ways of talking with the hands.

SEVEN
Conducting:
The leader's communication to performers

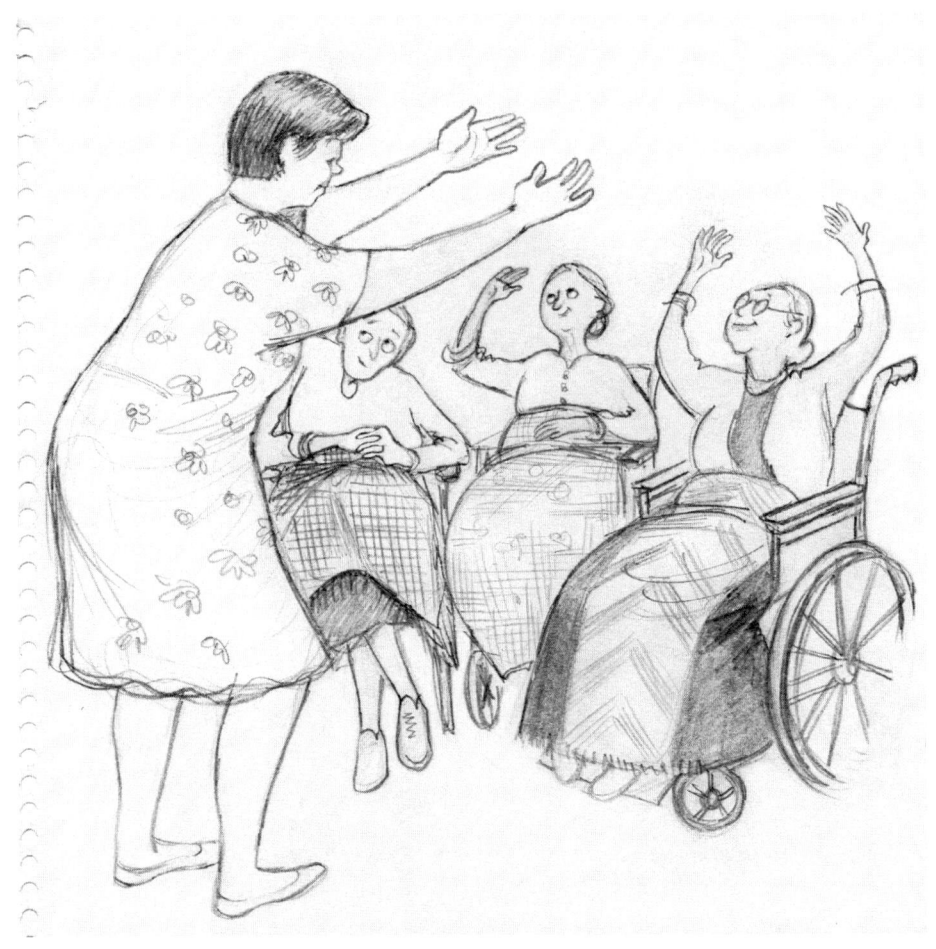

MUSIC & MOVEMENT
*When the activities assistant leads the group –
moving with music brings out the dancers in all of them.*

The five-week-old conductor

At first I felt a little shy to be so swiftly inside the walls and private life of complete strangers in Manhattan in a Stuyvesant Town apartment. As the young mother said on the phone, she was starting out with her first child born five weeks ago.

After I explained the lullaby project to both parents, Erika said her baby was just waking up. I could come into the bedroom to see her. On her back in the crib with pastel stuffed animals, her newborn daughter glowed with healthy beginnings.

"You want to see the change in her?" the new mother said as she started winding the music box mobile. Four animals danced on strings as the mobile turned. Tinkling sounds of "Raindrops Keep Falling on My Head" filled the quiet bedroom.

The baby started making sounds. As we watched from the doorway, Erika repeated her happy cries and cheers adding stage whispers to me, "See, she watches these things turn. She's conducting! She feels the music through her body. She's absorbing all of it. I'll let it stop for a few minutes and she'll start screaming."

We waited as the melody's notes faded and, sure enough, the infant started making restless sounds, fussing and sneezing. "She's waiting. I'll run back in and rewind it," Erika said. "Let's see how she changes when the music box goes back on."

When the music played again the baby's attention focused. She constantly worked her legs, walking on her back and making small outward thrusts with little fists.

"See, she does more leg work when she hears something." Gathering her beloved baby into her arms the new mother praised her, "Such a cutie! Yeah, musica!"

> This story can help us recall our own childhood – raising our children and grandchildren – the simplicity of sense memories and the intimacy and reassurance of loved ones in early relationships.
>
> What's your earliest or first musical memory?

Leader's Guide: Get everyone gently moving

In the following exercise, the leader of a group or an individual becomes a conductor of happy, familiar tunes. Classical music, such as Strauss' waltzes and Handel's "Water Music," provides rhythmic accompaniment.

Add arm movements. Imitate the conductor of an orchestra. Feel the changes in the music. Absorb all of it. Add vocal sounds – "whoooo–oooo, lay la, loooooo" – whatever you like that will stir the emptiness of the space you occupy with elders. Encourage your partner or group members to mirror your conducting by moving their arms with the music. Use a conductor's cue: "One, two, three and…"

This can be like cheerleading. Add batons, instruments or brightly colored, sequined and shiny movement scarves – anything that enhances the visibility of arm movements works.

Props like tongue depressors with sparkles glued on the end can accompany the anthem, "This Little Light." Have everyone join in the concert waving the shiny tongue depressors and singing the spirited tune that was made for conducting.

Add gentle rhythmic gestures, a light touch, a hug, a kiss and a kind word as you listen and move together.

Don't forget room-bound people.

Bring music boxes, small instruments and musicians to visit them.

Note the sparking lights in otherwise dim eyes, beaming smiles and nods.

The wheelchair conductors

The elders enjoy conducting music with graceful water movements that flow from their usual stationary postures in seats. One, sometimes two arms gyrate and spin, weaving almost visible scenes. Others look on, smiling and imitating our arm dances. Everyone enjoys mirroring movements.

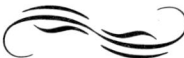

Anna is a retired music teacher. Using a toy maraca with streamers, she conducts a song with several new movements, ending the music with a bow and a flourish from her wheelchair. We notice that she is also able to carry on longer verbal exchanges since participating in musical activities.

Julia suffered a stroke and for many years has been able to speak in only short phrases. Softly she murmurs "lovely." She enjoys the music and responds with calm smiling facial expressions. I invite her to dance holding hands. We sway our arms together back and forth rhythmically.

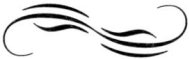

Laura has a hearing impairment. Yet she is still active and enthusiastic. She uses colored scarves to dance. She seems to hear the music better as we conduct the rhythms. There is a vibration – communication.

> Make it your purpose to stimulate conversations, deep caring and engagement. When men and women sit in isolated wheelchairs in front of TVs and at opposite ends of the halls, they can never discover the joy of connecting more deeply with each other.

Coaching spirits

    Be Sure…
        Your…
        Partners…See…Your Spirit Dancing Freely
            Feel…Your Energy Intimately…
            Listen…Sensuously…
        Spontaneously Embody…
        Embrace…
        Care About…
            What…You…Are…Doing…

EIGHT
Spontaneous songs:
The ordinary instinct of birds singing

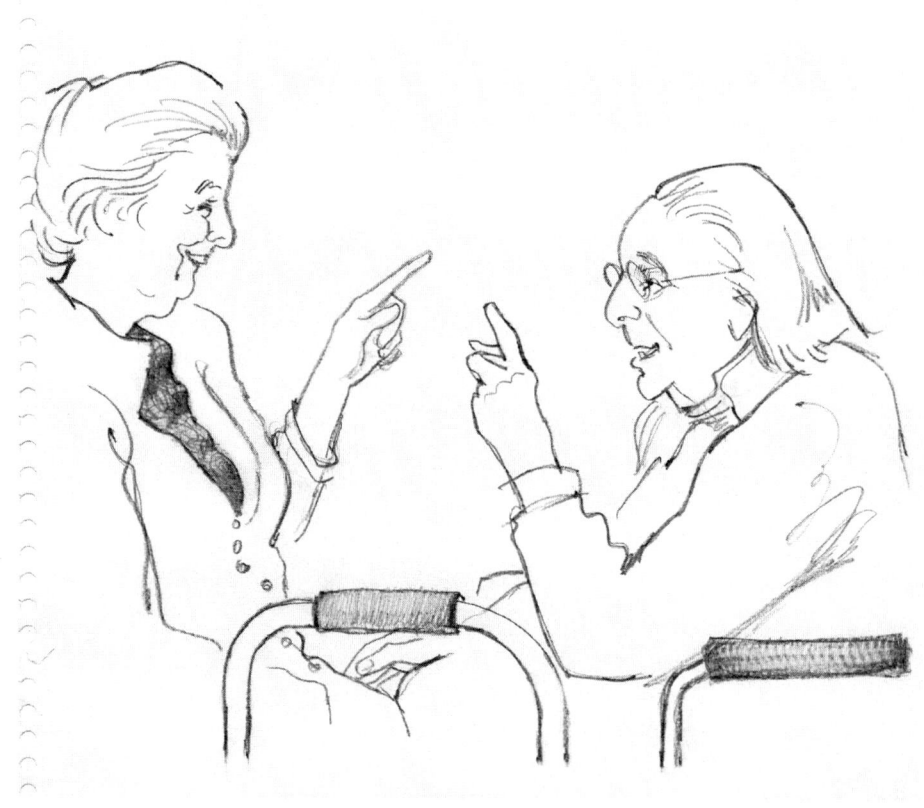

SISTERS' DUET
*When Carol and Gloria swap vocals and mirror movements,
they feel free as the birds.*

Sisters' duet

My neighbor said she would introduce me to the woman from Santo Domingo who babysat for her younger child. She advised me not to bring the tape recorder on the first visit. She said they wouldn't understand why I wanted to record such an ordinary everyday activity.

A short rugged freckled woman with dark hair, Tammy was clutching foil-wrapped Alka Seltzers in her hand when I met her. She told me she had a headache. Her baby had been crying all night and kept her awake. I told her of my interest in ways of putting children to sleep. She said, "It's very hard to put the children to sleep. You have to try everything!" Last night her husband laughed at her. She said she was in the bedroom singing to her child who stood up in the crib looking wide awake and blowing spit bubbles.

Tammy preferred that we try recording her singing lullabies in the late afternoon because her three children often took naps in the parlor. When I went down the following day I had to wait outside the door a while before it was opened. I came through the curtain hanging between the short alcove and parlor and there was Jasmine half-dressed on the couch. Tammy rushed the two-year old back to the bathroom. We laughed at her innocence. Returning shortly, Jasmine smiled slowly. She stared at me and said my name is "Julia" not "Hulia" as Tammy calls me. Jasmine seemed to understand that I am not Spanish, therefore "J" is sounded as "J" in Jasmine.

The large living room was dimly lit – the shades pulled halfway down and the windows closed to keep the sound of city traffic low. The TV was on – children's shows and cartoon sounds in the background. Five-year-old Miguel was sitting in an upholstered easy chair with a TV table in front of him. Jasmine was in blue shorts now and right at my side on the couch. Nine-month-old Melody was in the yellow playpen. Tammy apologized for being busy in the kitchen a few minutes. Miguel wanted potato like his father who loves potato any time.

While I waited the two older children examined my bag that says "Music Is my Bag." When Miguel read "music" I questioned him and found out he didn't know the word but read the music symbols on the bag.

I showed them the recorder and started recording them talking and singing. Tammy and I sat on the couch with room for the kids between. They were like an octopus their legs and arms swimming over us. Tammy admitted she was not relaxed. The microphone kept getting knocked by the kids moving in and out of her lap.

However, when I played parts of the recording, the baby heard her mother singing and picked up her head. Her face shone alert and attentive to the sound of her mother singing the familiar lullaby coming out of the recorder. The two older children knew I put their mother's voice into the box. But something very naked, primitive and magical was available in the baby's response, like a brave turtle protruding its small head from the shell of darkness and innocence reaching for the assurance and comfort of her mother's voice.

Even though there was all this chaos of TV and busy kids in the room, whenever Tammy sang a lullaby, it would all fade out. The spell of her singing would quiet and calm the room. The song was a beautiful blossom that filled the room as long she sang it, confidently, securely.

Her children were growing up singing with each other. At their mother's feet the sisters knelt facing each other. Jasmine started playing with sounds expressing hums, glides, trills and smacks to her baby sister. When the older girl changed the sound, the baby repeated her new sounds. Mirroring facial expressions, the sisters locked into this duet all their own.

> This story can be used to focus on daily celebrations and the richness of intergenerational relationships. What is your favorite memory of a childhood duet? Who were you with? What was the conversation about?

Leader's Guide: Rhythm sharing

This activity offers both the caregiver and caregetter an enjoyable sensory experience. The leader helps the elders to imitate rhythms and sounds.

Cut material into three-inch-wide yard-long strips. The number of strips will depend on the number of people and the group's abilities to partner with each other.

Demonstrate rhythm sharing with a partner:
> Face your partner and hold the strip with one hand.
> Pass it behind your partner's back at the waist.
> Grasp the strip with your other hand.

You now are ready to rock your partner gently while you make soothing sounds – sighs, moans, groans, sobs, howls, cries, hums, drones, purrs, murmurs, trills and whispers. You may speak softly, exhale noisily, enjoy joyful musical care and sing a song to your partner. Give your partner the feeling of swinging in a hammock or cradle. Feel one rhythm together. Your partner will enjoy being rocked and soothed for a few minutes.

Now take a turn being rocked by your partner.

Help everyone to find partners. Encourage them to imitate gently the rhythm sharing activity with each other, taking turns being rocked and sung to.

Adapt this activity for people who use a wheelchair. If it is impossible to slide a strip of material behind a person, dance with the person in the wheelchair gently to give the enjoyable sense of movement and rhythm.

Elders' duets

For agitated or restless elders, the first thing I do is sit at their level and talk to them.

Julia likes to clap her hands. If she is clapping very fast, crying or quarreling, I will start clapping and talking softly at her pace. I slow down – gradually transferring both of us to a quieter rhythm.

Often, just talking makes the transition to a calmer pace. Sometimes I will open my mouth and start to sing. The others join in, relaxing.

Christina rotates her head more, gently greeting others with a brightened smile. Gloria rocks her right leg and foot, passing the yellow sensory foam ball directly to Denise. Gloria and Denise volley with each other for about a minute. I am sure the change in the mood has to do with vibrations of the voice, literally bringing us together.

At an Italian senior center, a grandmother confides, "Sometimes when a couple is making love and the fellow dozes her to sleep, he says '*Nonna nonna* my darling – go to sleep my darling.'" *Na, na – ninna–nanna – nonna – nonnarella* – are soothing sounds from the Italian baby language used in lullabies.

Looking knowingly around at all the other grannies gathering at my tape recording session, she chuckles, adding in a hushed voice, "She closes her eyes under passion of love."

> You're never too old to smile, to quiet another or yourself,
> to remember love and to live until you die.

Coaching spirits

Have a lullaby conversation:
    Listen to…The sounds…
    Imitate them…Introduce new sounds…
    Take turns…

When you sing…
    …leave time for the person to repeat
        …each part of the song
    …echo the voice you hear singing to you
        …put words clearly out
        …fly them like clouds in the air like rainbows
        …let the other person watch
            your mouth…
            your lips…
            your teeth…
            your eyes…
            your mind…
            your thoughts…
            closely…

NINE
Greetings:
Familiar calls from long ago

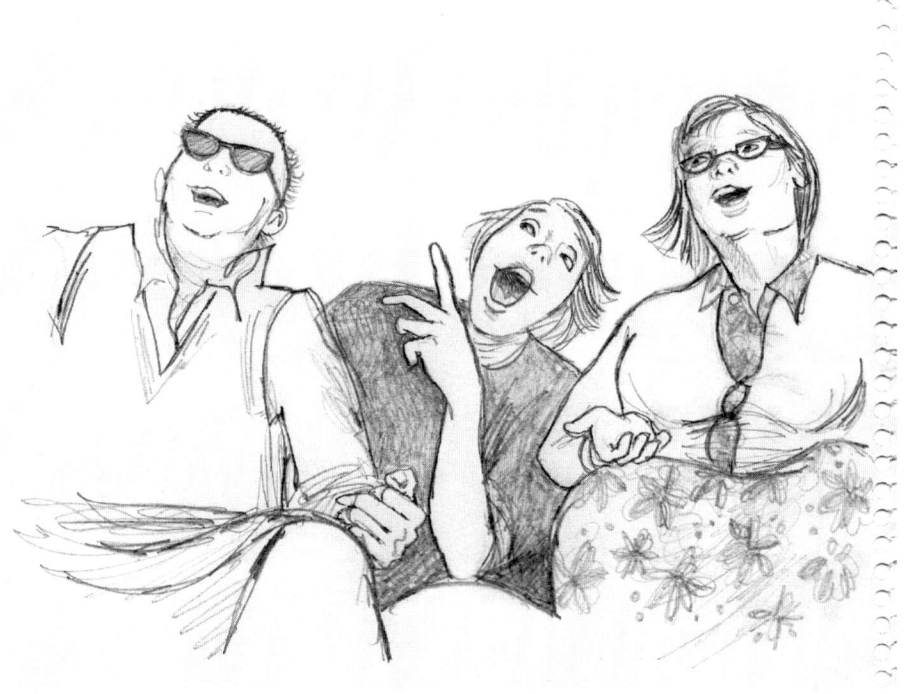

ROBERT, CONNIE AND BARBARA
*Names and common greetings engage people
in recalling lively moments of their lives.*

Bedtime calls

In Jackson Heights, Isabel leans out the window. "Did you leave the green door open?" she calls to her four-year-old son playing on the path below.

"Gerr-ie, Gerr-ie, time to come inside, soon…." She sings many times before the boy finally arrives.

They do their bedtime rituals – brushing teeth, washing face, finding pajamas, reading a story together. His favorite story, "Hansel and Gretel," matches the Dutch look of the neighborhood's red brick four-story houses. After a few pages, Gerrie starts flying around the apartment half-naked and making bird cries. His mother insists now he must "*Go to bed!*"

When he lands in bed, Isabel lies down next to him and cuddles, trying to get him to calm down. He babbles on since they really haven't talked all day. Isabel is tired, her voice a low warbling like a soothing cello behind his constant jabber. Then she sings. After another song and a loving backrub, she joins me in the parlor.

"You're talking too loud!" Gerrie calls as we start to talk. Then he wants to know what to dream about. He complains that he always dreams of what *she* says, but he cannot dream about what *he* says. Isabel answers and assures him every time that she is still there and they are home together in the darkness.

As Gerrie falls asleep, Isabel recalls her aunt who said she needed a second cup of coffee to get her children through bedtime. "Putting everyone to bed is such a job!" Isabel says and points to the toys strewn all over the room and the hallway waiting to be cleaned.

"The children sleep so loud," she sighs as she gets up to bring Gerrie the glass of water he is requesting. "At last there is peace in the house."

> This story can help us recall the voices of our childhood as well as all the things we do before we go to bed and fall safely asleep. Do you recall any children's games that included calls and responses, such as tag, hide and seek, bingo?

Leader's Guide: Lullabies with childhood memories

Lullabies are often characterized by descending tones accompanied by the soft sound of a rattle, a rocking chair or a cradle. This activity draws on deeply stored but still warm memories of lullabies to awaken a spontaneous chorus.

It is easy to get back to spontaneous songs. Start by playing with falling tones.

Introduce pitch by singing high, "This is Momma Bear," and then singing low, "This is Papa Bear." Sing the names of the elders using two notes. Go from high to low, or if you have a piano play the notes D then B.

Ask the elders to recall the ways their mothers and fathers called them. Lead a discussion using these questions.
- Did your parent shout, say or sing your childhood names?
- Why were you being called?
- What was your response to being called by your parent?
- What kind of a person was your parent?
- What did you call your parent?
- When did you call for your parent?

Ask how their mothers said or sang their names when they were putting them to sleep or when they were calling them for dinner. Likely, these will include a distinct singsong lilt.

Everyone enjoys remembering when they were loved – as well as when they knew they were in trouble!

Remembering childhood calls

Retirees Robert and John sing their childhood names – "Bob-by," "John-nie."

Millie remembers her mother's nickname for her, "Beav-er." The oldest in the group, Carol who is in her nineties, remembers where she was when her mother called her home and what she was doing. This leads to relaxing reminiscences about childhood games.

We talk about singing games with children and singing for ourselves at home. Athena moved from Florida to Brooklyn. Her musical interests have changed from spirituals to Caribbean music. She wants to play her flute more by ear.

Larry remembers songs from the military with doggerel verses. Barbara's husband talks about his Irish family singing while he hid under the table blocking his ears. His dentist sings Johnny Mathis tunes.

Barbara is unable to carry a tune. She hears high notes better than low. But her life is a musical. She knows many songs even if she cannot reproduce what she hears. She has songs of her own.

John talks about his happy childhood with six siblings. "Oh, Danny Boy," is his favorite song because it names Danny, a child who died whom John remembers with love.

> There is power in our narratives. Everyone has a different story to tell or not to tell.
>
> Perhaps only feeling together and being together is the power of our lifelong narratives.

Coaching spirits

Have you noticed the bells signal?
Stopped your work… thankful…
Lifted your face…smiled… heard the simple tones…
Put down your burden… like a peasant at Matins…
Called… Told by a more… ancient voice….
Have you pondered… witnessed… the love… with faith…
Believed more than words can tell…
Here?

TEN
Humming:
Meaningful murmurs of living

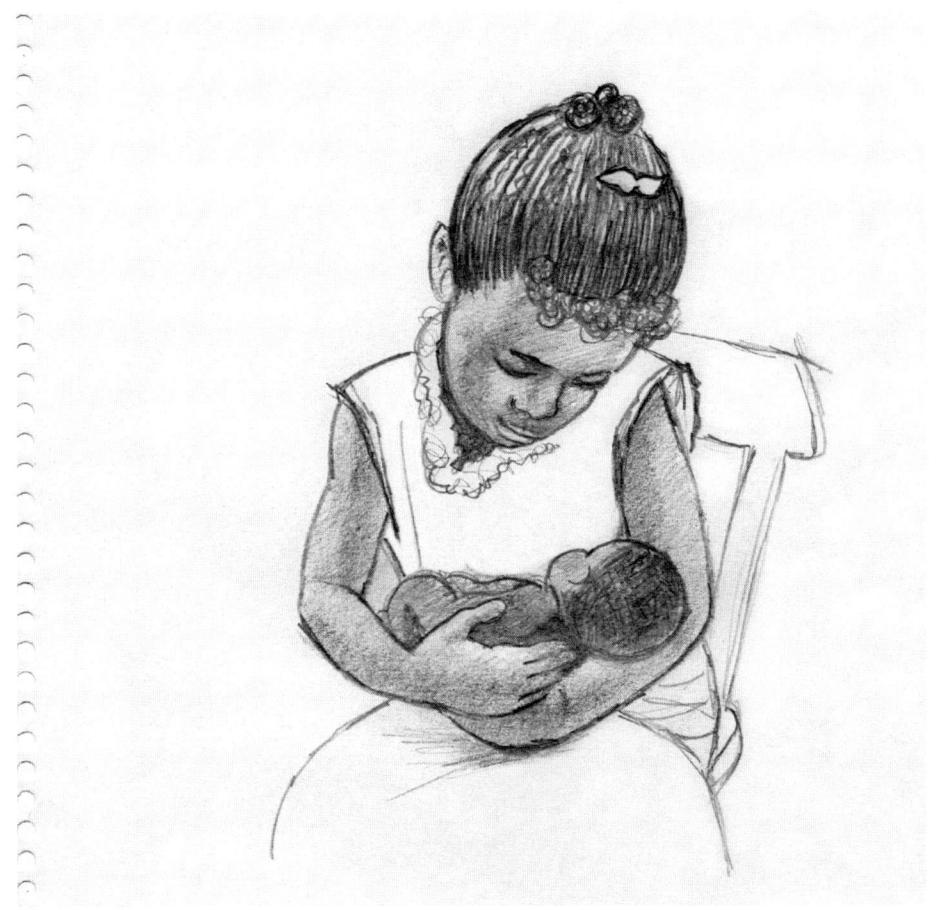

RUBY AND DOLLY
"There is a song in everything."
(Me-dee-kes, a Native American of the Tsimpshean tribe)

The humming mother and mosquitoes

When mothers sing they do not sing only the words. They take the baby's babbling sounds and improvise. A lullaby often starts with melodious babble. No words, only humming. Mothers may calm down overexcited children by stroking their faces, arms and legs.

Humming and crooning sounds make comforting, rhythmic and soothing music. A mother shared the birdlike humming that her Ukrainian mother gave her as a child.

This young mother got the idea to try to fool her six-week old baby into sleeping. She directed me to pull the bedroom shades and throw certain covers and diapers on the bed. She lay on her side beside the little baby on the big bed.

"I love to sleep, but this is a hard one," she commented playfully as she started humming a repetitive sound like waves hitting the shore – like the loon's beautiful mournful call – "OOO-ooo, OOO-ooo, OOO-ooo…" I felt myself relaxing hypnotized by this woman's continuous insistent aural presence.

"Lu lee, lu lee," she whispered her sweet Ukrainian "night-night."

The baby almost was tricked into sleep but her mother had to readjust the situation moving the pillow a few times. The baby started fussing and crying. Up the shade went. Immediately the baby was quiet, wide-eyed with the daylight like a wonder waking us all.

A Chinese artist once told me that he thought the real first lullaby is by mosquitoes. He said, "I remember when I was one year old and a lot of mosquitoes were flying on top the netting over me."

He hummed to illustrate then continued – "After a while they were very strong and made me sleep because of the blood in the body like a river running. Same kind of harmony of the sounds floating, floating, floating with the blood becomes the same rhythm with the blood and that's what makes us comfortable."

This Asian father also told me that in order to collect real lullabies I would have to go into rural China. When I asked him why, he explained that in China many places do not have any television, or movies or radios. The lullaby becomes very, very delicious, very important.

He said China is a very big country. There are a lot of mountains and rivers and little villages. Each village has a different kind of lullaby because lullabies are influenced by the wind blowing in the villages. Some winds blow very strong. Some are murmuring.

"Have you ever seen the dance in Hawaii?" he asked me.

"The dance is very soft hula-hula dance because the wind, the island breezes blow that way. Here in New York City if the mother is singing to the baby, suddenly the telephone rings! The lullaby is destroyed by the telephone ring. The lullaby singing must be intimate, only friend to friend, or lover to lover, or mother and child, very close and secure."

When he was six years old, he slept in his mother's arms. He said: "That is why I have sensitive feelings. When I was young, she gave me sensitive feelings through her lullabies."

Lullaby in Chinese is *yao lan chu*. *Yao* means "basket." *Lan* means you push it. A lullaby is a small song, *chu*, very individual, very private as long as the voice is very direct.

> This story helps us rediscover the musical and intuitive healing powers of our natural voices. Singing inward makes it easier for the caregiver and those in pain to release their suffering and breathe more deeply channeling healing and transition.

Leader's Guide: Something everyone can do!

Start by humming waves. Use the "m" sound. Try to use a lot of space in your body. Open up your voice and relieve tensions. Once humming gets started, it just makes itself up. Bounce the humming sound around. Try not to think of what you are doing. Repeat your hums, or vary them.

To introduce humming to a partner or group, say:
   Humming is like a wave.
   It's a flowing.
   It just goes up, (hum "m" up a few tones)
   and down, (hum "m" down a few tones)
   up, and down, (hum "m" up a few tones, hum "m" down a few tones)
   up, and down. (hum "m" up a few tones, hum "m" down a few tones)
   If you look at a wave long enough, it will put you to sleep.

Skywrite together: Use your arms and fingertips to trace a wave going up and down, changing the length and height of the waves for variety as you hum up and down the scales.

Use your arms and body movement to keep the rhythm and hold attention. Get close to your partners, go to their level, and use your touch to establish rhythms.

Don't be shy about going on for longer than you thought possible. Humming can become meditative and create a blanket of harmony for everyone involved.

Your spontaneous voice is enough, but if you have a piano or instrument, play the simple melody line of a familiar song such as "Rock-a-bye Baby" or "Hush Little Baby."

Once the group has the melody, encourage everyone to hum.

Pause between songs for gentle probing. Ask for suggestions of other favorite songs. Ask if anyone knows the words or get everyone to join in on humming rounds of "Row Row Row Your Boat."

Conclude with everyone humming the same song.

> This activity is especially good for people who are too weak to sing and emotionally remote in advanced stages of dementia. Humming is something everyone can do!

Mmmmmmmm – they're all thoughts

An African-American mother passes on her Southern heritage to her daughter. She shares memories of her hometown:

"In Georgia, there were a lot of old-lady sounds. There were certain hums and grunts that they did that I also notice across cultures and across ages. My grandmother used to rock on the porch. She would communicate like that. You say something to her and she would go *'mmmmmm'* – sort of half-talking and half-humming. I often communicate that way with people. Humming seems like a universal language. Often in my New York City neighborhood I'll relate to older women that way. They know exactly what I'm talking about! I do that at the end of the day to ease myself out. It's a series of thinking and making sounds and listening to them – but they're all thoughts."

"New York City Lullabies" CD, Track 3 "Hummings"

> Simply relaxing together, nodding and sighing is responsive caregiving.
>
> "…She softened, took my hand and asked how I was doing." From "A Patient's Story" by Kenneth B. Schwartz of The Schwartz Center for Compassionate Healthcare
>
> Small gestures are very powerful and can bring much needed moments of calm to the apprehensive sufferers of illness and memory loss who feel warmed by your presence.

Coaching spirits

A lullaby is like a wave…
    Like a thought…
        If you're very peaceful…
            You can send your peace…
                Through the sounds…
                    To other people…

Like some people hold…
    Other people's hands…
        And do not say words…
Just send the love to other people…

    A lullaby is a small song…
        Very individual…
        Very private…
            As long as the voice carries…
                Like a wave…
                    A beautiful lovely love sound…

ELEVEN
Communications of love:
Touching is language is singing is dancing

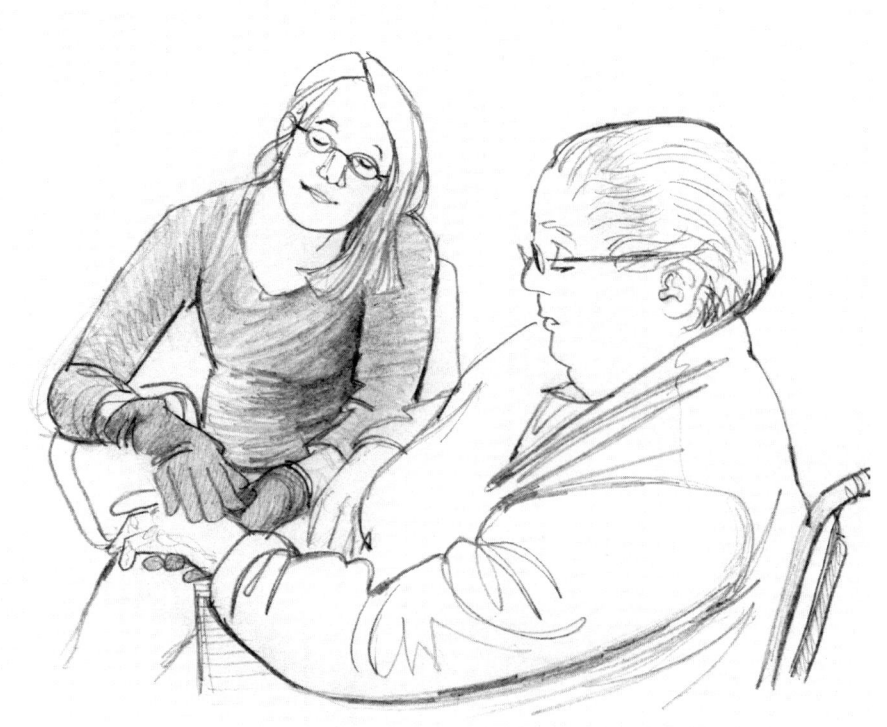

MARCIA AND BETTY
The power of love is ageless and timeless.

Simple human touch

Bedtime often signals the return to the oneness of the womb for both the mother and the child. In the womb it was all one – sound, smell, taste, touch. We guide our children into womblike feelings of safety using lullabies. Sometimes touch is the only way to communicate with a care recipient. Through gentle loving touch, you can say a lot.

In New York City, I visited a mother who wanted a rocker but had no room for one in her small apartment. She sat on the edge of the straight-backed chair rocking, responding to her baby's sounds and wiggles. Over and over during this visit, I was aware that this mother was like a sorceress and an improviser constantly looking for what works, and sticking with that.

I could see her rocking from her roots, first sideways, then without a change in beat, shifting the rocking to a back-and-forth dipping. What a dancer this mother was with her infant at her breast. Her total involvement was intimate like the words of a lullaby that poet Federico Garcia Lorca found in Spain: "Lullaby, my child, oh we will build a hut in the country and go inside. We must make ourselves smaller, tiny, and the walls of the little hut will touch our skin. We must live in a tiny place. If we can, we will live inside an orange, you and me. Even better inside a grape."

She was feeling what the baby needed and repeating her tiny sounds. "We're both sopranos!" she whispered. I kept checking the LED lights on the level meter to see what kind of sound I was getting. She said she always sings softly because she wants her child to be a relaxed girl – not a nervous wreck.

> "These acts of kindness – the simple human touch from my caregivers – have made the unbearable bearable. The rulebooks, I am sure, frown on such intimate engagement between caregiver and patient. But maybe it's time to rewrite them."
>
> From "A Patient's Story" by Kenneth B. Schwartz

Leader's Guide: Soothe! soothe! soothe!

To lead this activity with one other person you will need soothing aromatic hand lotion and/or a basin for washing hands.

Begin by eliminating any competing noises. Shut windows and doors and turn off the television. Select calming background music that invites humming or singing. You may want to settle down yourself by clapping and patting your hands, legs and arms – yawning – breathing deeply and exhaling sssssssssss and zzzzzzzzzzz. When you feel relaxed, gently take your partner's hand in both of your hands. Hold it to let both of you get used to the touch. Watch for any negative feedback such as reluctance to let you hold hands or clenching of fists. If there is hesitation say, "That's okay, maybe later," and move on to others.

Slowly caress and continuously move your hands, massaging the hand while moving from fingertips upward toward the wrist. Focus your attention and loving intention on your partner. You may want to hum and sing a favorite song together.

> A playful game helps two people get in touch with each other's energy and movement. Sometimes I add an exercise called "The Finger Dance" created by Arthur Hull to hand massages and music sessions.
>
> "May I have this dance?" I ask. Martin's blue eyes brighten. He is laughing aloud when I stand in front of him and lightly touch his index finger to my index finger dancing with him. He leads then suddenly fakes exhaustion by collapsing his head and shoulders and dropping his hands into his lap with a loud sigh. Soon he is alert and ready for more. He turns to Sarah seated beside him in a wheelchair to continue finger dancing with a new partner.
>
> To finger dance with a partner:
>
> Touch your partner's index finger with your index finger and make casual paths in the air while the person's finger follows yours. Take turns leading and following. Close your eyes. Finger dance.

Connecting the eyes with the ears and the skin

Mary said her mother, who suffered from dementia, didn't have the words to respond to her or the family. Then one attendant in the nursing home talked to her mother differently than any of her relatives did, and she responded.

"There was just a different level of comfort that this attendant had than the rest of us." Mary remembered happily, "She even took my Mom's cheeks and pinched them together to make her have fish lips. I never would have thought to do that and look at her – she was enjoying it!"

In a similar setting, I was removing Helen's stockings when she told me about how lousy and depressed she was feeling.

"All that French food!" she complained about dinner. "Why don't they just cook some good American food!"

She talked about her loss of eyesight. "I never realized how much the eyes are connected with the ears. I don't feel like talking with anyone. I don't know if they are talking to me. They seem to ignore what I say."

"It was so dark today," she said sadly as we got her ready to go to bed.

Like Helen, newborn babies are blind and often live with shocked and stressed-out adults who do not communicate lovingly with them. Like Mary's mother and Helen, children who are just learning to listen and speak often don't know if someone is talking to them. They can't always hear or tell what people say.

The blindness of birth like the darkness of night brings on the desperate need for comforting words and feelings. The process of bonding with touch creates rest, safety and contentedness.

> Talking regularly with loved ones and patients about life, aging, illness, family, friends and children helps us make a personal connection to their triumphs and troubles and makes them feel acknowledged and accepted.

Coaching spirits

Often I sent my elderly mother little things I found on my walks along beaches and in the woods. I also affirmed these little love tokens with intentions written in my journals. I wrote this poem to accompany a tuft of white downy feathers I found on a Rhode Island beach and tucked into the folds of my weekly letter home. Its message applies to other objects and people for whom touch and imagination can renew connection to themselves, their loved ones and the world.

> Hold
> this feather in your hands.
> Let it soften the cracks, mend.
> Don't sew for a week. Don't read.
> Rest your strained eyes, close them.
> Close your eyes. Envision that bird's flight
> After it left its mother – well-plumed, solo, silent.
> Reaching wider for love –
> catching flowers,
> leaves,
> feathers,
> touching
> others
> with
> close
> a-
> bun-
> dance.

TWELVE
Patterns of light, sound, motion:
The breathing presence of energy that connects us

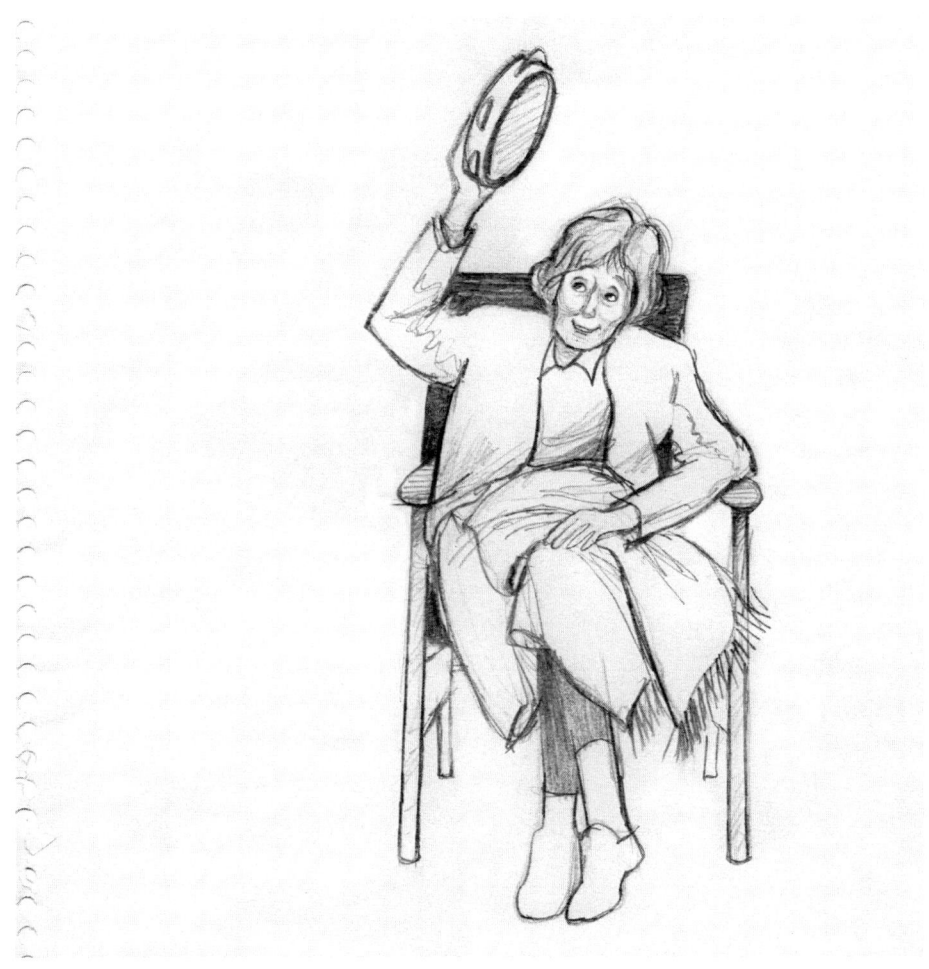

LILY WITH TAMBOURINE
Old age is what you make it!

Lois's colors

It often isn't easy to put aside the cares of the day. A lullaby or a story fills a child's mind with something different than ordinary preoccupations. A pattern – in Lois's case a visual pattern she created for herself – works the same way getting us out of our mundane existence into something else.

Lois, a New York City parent, told me about what used to put her to sleep as a child: "Do you know that if you close your eyes in a dark room you see tiny, tiny dots of color – red ones and blue ones – swimming colors going up and down, up and down. If I had my eyes open in an apartment with Venetian blinds I'd get the cars, the traffic moving against the patterns of the blinds. I can remember watching these patterns."

"I had games – I had contests with colors." Lois remembered the reds going one way, the blues and greens going another way. "I was a child who wanted a family. I was an only child. So even when I went to sleep I had to have lots of people in my world with me. The reds were a family, the greens were a family, the blues were a family. That was my fantasy."

"It wasn't a game," Lois recalled. "Blue was always my favorite color so the blues would always win, or the blues would stop and talk to me." Lois laughed at herself. "Actually it probably didn't put me to sleep. It probably kept me awake!"

> Colors also carry their own vibrations. I always wear bright colors when I visit the elderly in nursing homes. Bright colors can wake up the brain and stimulate brain activity. They help dementia patients who have been sidelined in wheelchairs break out of the "inactivity coma."
>
> From Christine Knowles reflections
> on *As Long as You Sing, I'll Dance*

Leader's Guide: Chanting lulling syllables

In many lullabies, patterns are repeated to create an almost hypnotic effect. "Lull" means to soothe to sleep or quiescence by imitating the repetition of lu-lu, la-la, lullay, or similar sounds appropriate to singing a child to sleep.

Lullaby sounds are like drumbeats heard and internally felt. They can connect us back to the first sounds every human hears inside the womb – the mother's heartbeats. This sense of the nurturing connection to the mother ensures trust and safety so the child can go to sleep.

Some of us remember the songs our mother used to sing at bedtime when we were children. We may not remember the words, but we know lots of love came through. What we remember best is how our parents use to murmur sweet nothings – *shh, shh – there there – sweetum – coochy coo – honey –* and other familiar sounds.

Languages are different. But it's like the Andrews Sisters sang in "Bei Mir Bist Du Schon":

"I could say *bella bella* even say *voonderbar*
Each language only helps me tell you how grand you are."

With lullabies, I could say *lu lu, la la*
Even say *ninna nanna,*
Do do, da da, shah shah, ma ma
Each language only helps me tell you –
I love you – rest, it's okay –
I am with you –

Sit beside or near your loved ones and those to whom you give care. Even when they are suffering and in pain or medicated, even when they are too tender to be touched or even when they are dying, you can soothe and comfort them with patterns of sounds. They will feel your breathing presence and know they are not alone and you are part of their life, giving care.

The familiar voice, the rhythmic words, the lulling repetitions lower the threshold of consciousness. One woman told me that her nanny would read recipes from a cookbook to her at bedtime. She found this catalogue of words helped clear her mind of non-restful thoughts.

If you need inspiration, open a telephone book and chant the names out loud. The alphabetical order gives the phone book's list of names an appealing rhythm and rhyme.

Remind everyone about falling asleep at night when they were children. Tell them:

"Julia remembers falling asleep at night. She would play with rhythms. Her mother and father would yell up the stairs, 'Julia, are you asleep yet?' and she would take that sentence and accent different syllables, singing herself to sleep:

Julia are you asleep YET?
JULIA are you asleep yet?
Julia are YOU asleep yet?
Julia are you ASLEEP yet?"

Take any sentence and accent a different syllable or word each time you say it.

Make the word louder and stronger. Listen for changes in rhythms, the feelings expressed, and new meanings.

Personalize this by addressing each member of the group with a different question, then chanting together. For example:

Billy, are you hungry YET?
BILLY are you hungry yet?
Billy are YOU hungry yet?
Billy are you HUNGRY yet?

The magic of imagination

I read the "Yes, Virginia" editorial to several elders at a community social hour. They listened attentively to the famous reply that the editor of the *New York Sun* wrote in 1897 to the letter from eight-year-old Virginia O'Hanlon who asked if there really was a Santa Claus. "Not believe in Santa Claus!" the audience recited the well known lines with me. "You might as well not believe in fairies."

The elders, some of them nearly 100 years old, chuckled and smiled.

A discussion followed after I finished reading. One cynical woman said, "It's about the imagination – the importance of it. As you get older like us, you lose your imagination along with everything else."

I asked Lewis if he heard this and did he agree. "Do you still use your imagination? You're an artist!"

Lewis responded – "The imagination is extremely important. I use my imagination when I am planning my art work." He did not agree with the skeptical elder who thought we lose our ability to imagine.

Laura, who is losing her eyesight and can no longer walk, called out in strong agreement with Lewis, "Mine is getting stronger!"

Just then a visitor who happened to be Laura's daughter walked into the room and up to our table. I questioned everyone: "Oh look who's here! Do you know who it is?"

"Peter Pan!" Laura joked. We all laughed with delight at her quick answer.

> Imagine a bucket of muck. You put your hand in and dig around in order to find a diamond. What does this diamond you find sparkling with light stand for in your life?
>
> What nourishes you emotionally and spiritually?
>
> How can you take care of your diamond, nurture it so it continues to give you beauty?

Coaching spirits

When his baby had an operation, the new father chanted to the Kuan Yin Bodhisattva who is known as the "Regarder of the Cries of the World" (in the West she is the "Goddess of Compassion and Mercy" or the Holy Mother.) He said chanting to Kuan Yin calmed him down because he felt that this was the only tool he had to make their minds one.

As I listened to his chanting, I heard another voice affirming the emotional power of the human voice saying:

You are the sound you make in a way…
    Tune into the sound well…
        You will come from a real deep place…

The song makes our mind one…
    Takes away thought…
        Chanting forces you to deal with your breath differently…
            To come from a real deep place…
                Keeps you calm too…

We can occupy the same deep space…
    Of love and pain together…
        The same space…
            The only tool you have to make our minds one…
                Is the sound you make to calm us down…

Come from a real deep place…
    Make our minds one…
        Take away thoughts…
            You are the sound you make…

THIRTEEN
There's rhythm everywhere: Sharpen your personal communication style with gestures

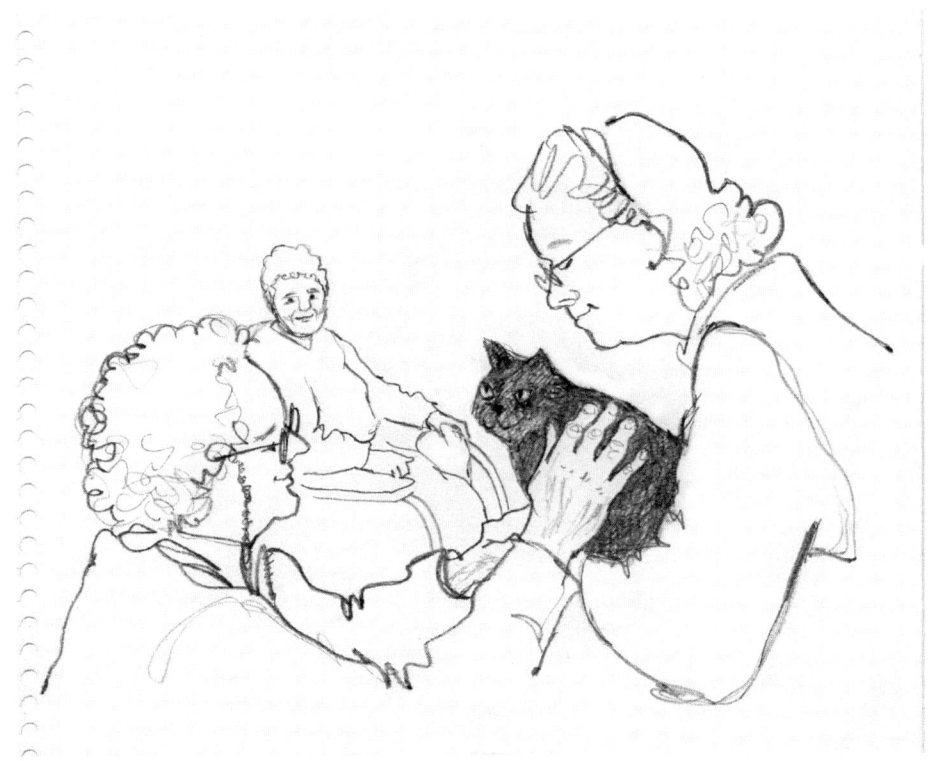

Max the Cat Visits
Everyone gathers around Max the therapy cat.

"La linda manita"

Because movements and gestures help us to connect to one another, they expand our communications. A Puerto Rican mother teaches her child in New York City the parts of the body with playful children's songs in Spanish.

"La linda manita" she sings turning both hands side to side, *"que tien el bebe."* (What pretty hands baby has.)

"Bump! Bump! Bump!" she continues, imitating the sounds and motions of crushing garlic in the *pilon* (mortar and pestle) and teaching her child a way of preparing the *sofrito* used in Puerto Rican dishes.

The song goes on to name other parts of the body like the nose, mouth, eyes and head by pointing *"el dedito"* (the finger) and ends with a flourish of hands and motherly cheers – *"Ay–yay–yay–yay–yay mi cabecita* (head)" teaching the characteristic body movements of salsa dance and flamenco and the traditional Puerto Rican way of talking with the hands. Re-animating your body and voice is like plugging into a circuit you may not have used in a long time.

> This story can stimulate recall of the nonverbal ways we all can communicate our love, compassion, hope and engagement with others.

Leader's Guide: Harriet the monkey

Biologists remind us that we can solve our problems by looking at the natural world. Inspirations from nature can help us communicate better. Modern and ancient codes of morality, society and culture contrive to lock us into prisons and cages so the zoo that is society can be organized. Yet we have minds. We can use them to make our own natural gestures.

In *The Year of the Gorilla*, George B. Schaller writes: "Animals are better observers and far more accurate interpreters of gestures than man." I have ample reason to believe this because I witnessed first-hand the ways of a monkey when I worked several years for a woman who suffered a terrible car accident that left her paralyzed from the neck down. Joanie lived in her Manhattan apartment with a simian aide from a therapy animal program called Helping Hands.

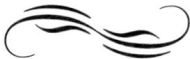

Helping Hands, a national not-for-profit corporation, breeds, raises and trains capuchin monkeys to assist severely disabled individuals with their daily activities. These affectionate, responsive companions are provided free of charge. In fact, I was losing my job as a nurse companion to a seven-pound capuchin monkey named Harriet.

Joanie raved about how much mental development and intelligence is dependent on physical ability. I could barely keep up with her simian aide. When Harriet stood on the table, we all raved, "She's so big!" We were amazed at how she stretched her agile arms and tail. Joanie had to remind us: "She *is very* small. I think she just looms large in our minds."

In my nursing chores, I used rhythm to survive like a monkey in a jungle. I learned these rhythms from living with this monkey in New York City. I practiced rhythms with Harriet – snapped my fingers, rapped on her cage door, hooted monkey style to call her back from her wild tirades.

Harriet used rhythmic sounds to calm herself – rapping with a block of wood like a woodpecker banging on a tree. When Joanie shouted, "Cage!" the monkey ran up and down our legs and laps over chairs and feet into her cage slamming the door behind her.

On rare occasions she cuddled in my arms like a baby. We rewarded her with green grapes and bananas. After peeling a half of one banana, she took it to some place in the living room. I sat on the couch. She returned with my pink socks. She carried them in her hands to the mirror and sat sideways with the piece of banana wrapped in my pink socks eating happily.

Later she sat in front of the mirror folding the socks inside-out. While I watered the plants she wiped up the floor with them. I put them in the cage with her to keep her company. This monkey had ways of animating the most trivial things and making great comedies of our lives as humans.

Sometimes Harriet was very sweet to visitors, coming to them curling in their laps right away, purring and chattering. Other times she got into playing. She did high jumps, springing and flying at me and landing on my shoulders or I was on all fours lunging at her and making surprise sounds. She loved it and wanted more and more. She chased me as I crawled and she rode on my back like a baby monkey in the jungle again. I asked her to swing under my belly. She swung on my arm and snorted in my armpit and sucked my neck and my ankle bone. I was the trees, branches, winds, coconuts that she missed. I was her jungle.

Joanie also developed many new gestures with her right arm, head and facial movements after Harriet came to live with her.

Let Harriet be your spontaneous caregiver guide!

Think of a mouthful of glistening white teeth, two fangs, the jungle and a tribe of her siblings. Then we see all we miss. Her excited gestures are gestures for meeting and reassuring kin monkeys. She is not a pest. She needs to be groomed and touched. By nature this is what she expects.

Now envision yourself inhabiting the body of a monkey. Think of yourself with a mouthful of glistening white teeth, two fangs – in the jungle with a tribe of siblings. We may have forgotten the vines, the soft ground, the swinging in the branches, excitement of rushing through the forest, but we have these remaining gestures. To understand her is to view her as part of her species rather than a member of the human system that has trapped her, tamed her and made her an orphan. We have these gestures of greeting and reassuring in common with the monkey, the dog, the fish, the birds and other fabulous natural creatures.

> "Generally, when threatened or upset, one first looks to others, wishing to engage their faces and voices and to communicate one's feelings to secure collective safety. These are called attachment behavior. Attachment is virtually the only defense young children have, as they cannot usually protect themselves by fighting or fleeing."
>
> Peter A. Levine, *In An Unspoken Voice: How the Body Releases Trauma and Restores Goodness*

Max the cat visits

As the activities director at a retirement community, I invited Deb and her therapy cat Max to visit many times. In fact, after the first time, nurses and other staff members in care plan meetings often named a "Max the Cat Visit" as an intervention for our aging, suffering residents. Just seeing Deb pushing Max in his stroller down the hallway brightened the day for our residents and staff.

Max exuded charm – two full-moon blue eyes surrounded by a shining long black lion's ruff. Max calmed the room like a serene night in a Rousseau painting. Every one wanted a look at him and several people lined up to hold

Max in their lap for just a moment.

One frail retired Sister of the Sacred Heart in skilled care was especially animated by Max's visits. The black feline curled in her lap purring under frail stroking fingers.

Memories of other cats and pets were recalled and shared long after the pleasures of Max the cat's visit.

> Provide something for your care recipients to hold on to. This means that you are making a nurturing contact.
>
> "Dance the mother of all dances — the dance of attachment…. We show our pleasure by gestures, smiles, tone of voice, a hug, a playful smile, by the suggestion of a joint activity, or simply by a twinkle in our eyes."
>
> From *Hold On to Your Kids*
> by Gordon Neufeld and Gabor Maté

Coaching spirits

I often listened carefully to my mother in the early stages of her dementia. One night as we returned home, she was enchanted by the red moon sinking low in the western sky. We stood together in darkness watching for a long time at the back door.

She recalled that red moon the next day. "Did you see it? Must be burying something, or someone," she said. Then looking at the calendar she became engaged in deep thought.

"The moon was burying a few days," she said with certainty, making sure that I was listening to her. "The moon is not always there. It hides sometimes."

When I asked her if it was the new or old moon – she knew it was the new moon, although she could not answer the correct year or month. The native ways of counting and observing are still sharp, although the brain damage of dementia causes loss of socialized learning and language.

The moon moves more quickly than any other planet in the sky. The moon never looks the same two nights in a row. Yet how many of us pause to observe and interpret as my aging mother did the many moons' luminous changing gestures?

Understanding the simplicity with which persons who are memory impaired can look at things gives you a better understanding of how to approach sensitive and humane caregiving.

PART THREE

Traditions

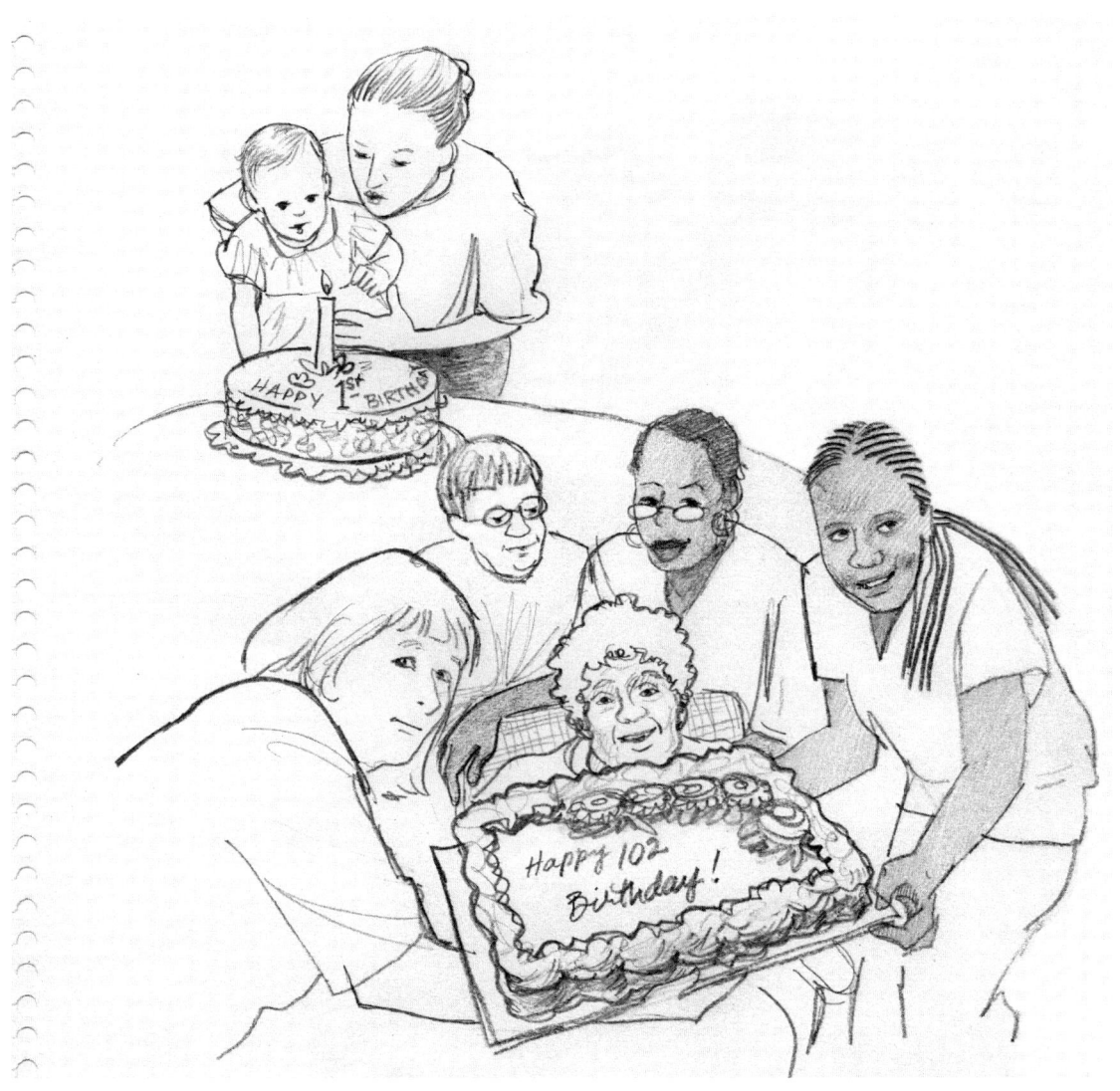

ANYA'S 1st & FRIEDA'S 102nd BIRTHDAYS
with their caregivers beside them.

FOURTEEN
Participatory chant:
The comfort of a storytelling circle

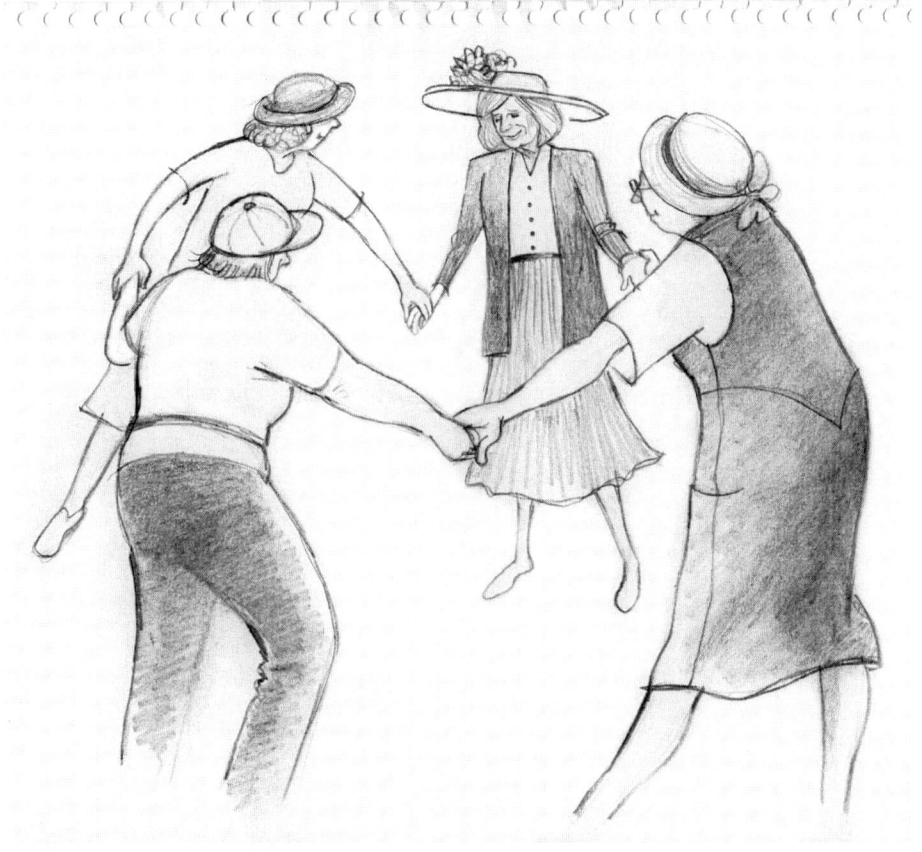

GARDEN PARTY CIRCLE DANCE
The sense of movement and rhythm is retained longer than most abilities.

A story of creation

I use routines of collecting during the day – connecting before and after breakfast, late afternoon, after an episode, holding hands in a circle saying yes, yes, yes – singing together while we gather for a program.

"Kumulipo" is a Hawaiian chant that tells a story of creation. It is 2,000 lines long. Parents recite it over a newborn to help bond the child to all other living things, those who came before and those yet to come.

In a similar way, a mother uses her daughter's name to create a lullaby.

"Susan Andromeda Miller has three names
Susan, **for your** mommy's family
Andromeda, **for your** African nation
Miller, **for your** daddy's family
Susan Andromeda Miller, has three names"

Andromeda is a Greek name composed of the elements that mean "to think like a man/warrior." Andromeda is the name of the daughter of Kassiopia who was to be sacrificed to the sea monster Medusa but was rescued by Perseus. Andromeda is said to have been an Ethiopian princess and ancient Ethiopians considered her and Perseus to be the progenitors of the black race.

> "Attachment rituals, fueled by this collecting instinct, exist in many cultures. The most common is the greeting which is a prerequisite for all successful intervention."
>
> From *Hold On to Your Kids*
> by Gordon Neufeld and Gabor Maté

Leader's Guide: Aloha greeting

The Aloha Greeting attempts to access the true wonderful comfort meaning of "aloha" that is much more than a word of greeting or farewell.

In this exercise ask each person to think and send good feelings to the others. To lead the chant, you will call on participants to name familiar beloved people, places and objects. Then incorporate their words into the group's rhythmic "Aloha" greeting. The group's words become a chant with vibrations and good feelings.

Introduce the word Aloha.
Leader: "Today, let's take time to greet each other, and share our breath with the Hawaiian word, aloha, which means *hello*, and *love* and *to share breath*. Aloha!"
Participants: "Aloha!"

Next play with the word a bit, breathing deeply and emphasizing the connection between the sounds of the word and the sound of the breath: "Ahhh…lowww…haaa."

Sometimes Hawaiians nod and actually touch their foreheads together as they meet saying first "Alo," then facing each other as they exhale the last syllable, "ha." This can provide a fun exchange of aloha spirits.

At the appropriate moment, the leader prompts a participant:
"Aloha, (participant's name). Give us the names of two relatives or people important to your life who we can greet."
Participant: "Marjorie and Johnny."

Together, the group uses these names and repeats the chant three times.
"Aloha, Marjorie and Johnny.
Aloha, Marjorie and Johnny.
Aloha, Marjorie and Johnny."

Leader: "Celebrate together! Aloha!
Let there be an echo to our song. One more Aloha!"
Participants: "Aloha!"

Continue the group chant with another question:
Leader: "What are two places where you find peace and strength?"
Participant: "<u>The chapel</u>."
Next participant: "<u>The community garden</u>."
Group: "Aloha, the chapel and community garden!"
Leader: "Celebrate together! Aloha!
Let there be an echo to our song. One more Aloha!"
Participants: "Aloha!"

Leader: "Tell us the names of the plants and animals on the earth useful to your life on earth."
Participant: "<u>Max the therapy cat</u>."
Next participant: "<u>Marigolds</u>, and <u>irises</u>."
Group: "Aloha, Max the therapy cat, marigolds and irises!"
Leader: "Celebrate together! Aloha!
Let there be an echo to our song. One more Aloha!"
Participants: "Aloha!"

Encore

Improvise lifting an imaginary glass, and toasting each other with "Cheers!"

Take turns around the group to give each person a chance to greet and toast the others.

"Down by the butternut tree"

You may be meeting an elder for the first time as a dependent human being. The value of hospice home care is that the caregivers go to meet people in the context of their whole lifetime and life style. There are usually pictures of loved ones, food and drinks offered and shared – significant clues about the whole spectrum of a person's existence. Some caregivers say they are walking on hallowed ground when they get to care for people in their own traditions at home outside the clinical setting. Look for clues that help you relate and communicate – stories, hobbies and reminiscences about both the living and the dead in order to give quality care. Here is an intimate portrait of an elder who inspired me with her wise traditions.

A mountain woman of French Canadian ancestry, Gram was one of the quiet hill folk. She lived alone in an old red farmhouse on the hill. She knew the mountain and told me where to find any bird, fish, flower or root of interest. Usually her directions began like this: "Down by the butternut tree…"

When I looked puzzled, she said, "Oh well. Of course you don't know where the butternut tree used to be. It was gone long before you came here!"

When I asked her to come along on hikes, she claimed nobody is older than she is so she could not go with me. I had to learn how to follow her stare out the window through the cherry tree over the railroad trestle up the beaver pond down to where the butternut tree used to be.

Her way of guiding did not so much include clear answers as it did generous clues. One time I arrived around dinnertime. The note written on paper with jagged edges hung from the silver chain of the kitchen ceiling lamp. "Up to the falls," it declared.

Before I followed this direction, I looked at a family picture on the fireplace mantle. Gram sat in the middle surrounded by three sisters and a brother. The women wore high-top boots and dark long-sleeved dresses. They were "big farm girls," as Gram said, "not slender pixies."

Before going to meet Gram in her favorite place I envisioned her sitting by the river, fishing pole in hand with her faithful dog nearby as I checked out her garden and found my work chore: currants ready to pick for jelly.

On the river road to the falls I met a little bent lady in a new dayglow orange cap, high rubber boots with a pole and a bag of tackle. She gave me a wink and a quick smile. "You're here! Isn't that just the berries!" Gram was already planning to put me to work in her currant bushes.

She made me want to keep her traditions, the ones she gathered from her grandmothers.

When she spread the afghan over one of her visitors napping on the couch, Gram said, "It's not for the birds." She whispered in the timeless mountain silence to an invisible presence, "My grandmother always covered someone over with a blanket when she went by."

Act as a compass point – orient – redirect.

Point out this and that. Find commonalities. We both have blue eyes. We both are wearing red today. Guide them in their new dependent role. Become an expert in the art of caregiving. Who could do better than you?

Coaching spirits

Get someone's attention before you speak to or touch her.
Be expressive with your face, gestures and whole body.
Keep doing the same thing over and over and over.
Counter your natural tendency to get louder.
Keep the sound the same (you just got louder!).
Use your hands to softly pat an even rhythm.
This gives a strong visual clue that focuses everyone's attention and unites the group.
Remind yourself to keep feeling loving.
Keep moving while you speak.

FIFTEEN
Praising with familiar kind words: The warmth of words

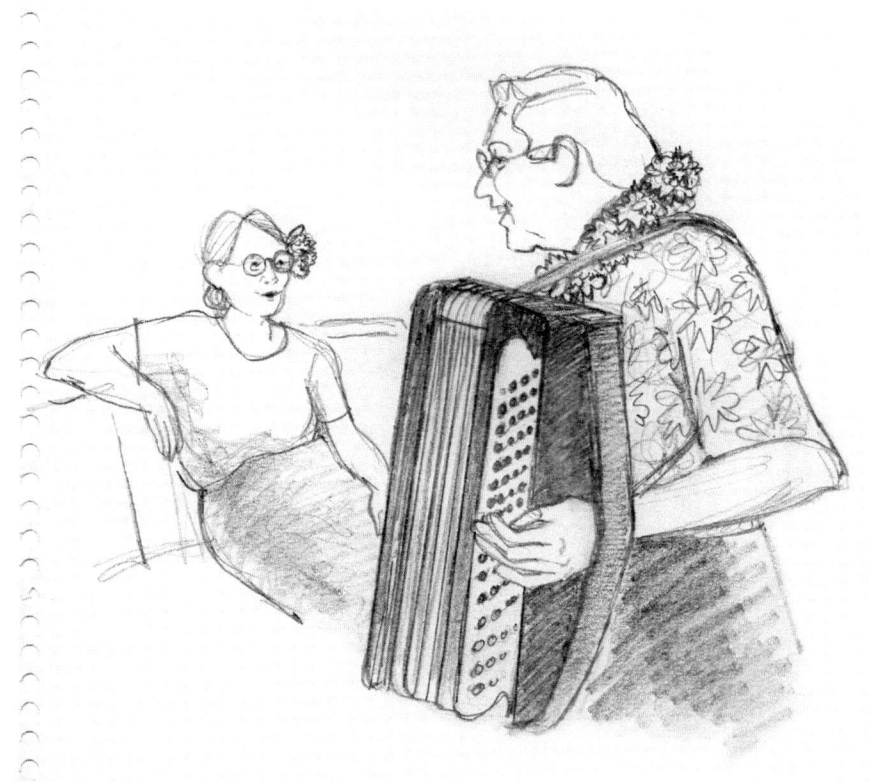

PANDY AND THE ACCORDION MAN
Make every hour sweet as a flower.

My carnation

Betty sat at the breakfast table. We talked about how pink her cheeks looked that day. She glowed as she remembered the story that her mother told her about walking by the river.

A village woman praised Betty – "Oh, what a pretty baby!" then playfully acted like she was going to take Betty out of her mother's arms. "I'm going to steal your baby away!" the woman teased.

Hugging herself tightly, Betty pretended to be her mother holding her infant close to her breast. She called out fiercely remembering her mother's passionate response, *"No, no! Mi carnacion!"* (No, no! My carnation!) She rocked herself back and forth quickly.

A few weeks later a fierce pneumonia took Betty suddenly away forever. She died over the weekend.

I stopped to buy flowers. Thoughts raced – *You're late for work – will they have carnations? It hit me again – where will I ever find one carnation to replace her? My carnation!"*

"My carnation!" I sang the words slowly as I studied the colors to select the exact pinks and glowing ambers of her rich complexion. The check-out-clerk looked at the cash register. She paused to question me as she read aloud, "Two for one, why not?"

I raced back and gathered another dozen – white, white dusted with pink, yellow, apricot, salmon, red, scarlet carnations. Carnations that blended together to create her brilliant unassuming face. *"My carnation!"* Her memories are now my memories.

Leader's Guide: Praise songs

Flowers are commonly used to praise the beauty of a baby. Parents say, "You are my rose" or "my carnation" in Spain, France, Italy, and Greece. "My tulip flower" is used in Persia. "Lily white" means "pretty" in China. "Pretty as a lotus" is a compliment in India. A mother in Syria sings, "You are pretty as basil in the garden."

Begin seated in a small circle. Greet and introduce the participants to each other. Talk about how good everyone looks today. For example: "What a pretty blue sweater, Evelyn!" "Barbara, you look so happy in your yellow sweat suit."

Praise each person through flower names describing qualities of color, smell, taste and touch.

Use the prompt, "You are my rose."

Follow with "You are crushed mint leaves carried in my mother's apron pocket."

And "You smell of her fresh summer garden."

Consider these mothers' special loving words.
From Corsica:
"You are sweetly-blowing savory,
You are thyme, smelling of incense,
Growing on Mount Basella, and on Mount Cassoni;
You are rock hyacinth on which the flocks feed."
Sings the Sicilian mother:
"Hush, child of my breath, bunch of jasmine,
handful of oranges and lemons."

Terms of endearment can be found in many familiar songs. Sing or read the following to help participants remember their own endearing terms in the lyrics of well-known love songs.

Song 1. "You Are My Sunshine"

You are my sunshine, my only sunshine
You make me happy when skies are gray
You'll never know, dear, how much I love you
Please don't take my sunshine away.

Song 2. "Let Me Call You Sweetheart"

Let me call you sweetheart, I'm in love with you
Let me hear you whisper that you love me too
Keep the love light glowing in your eyes so true
Let me call you sweetheart, I'm in love with you!

Song 3. "Daisy, Daisy"

Daisy, Daisy, give me your answer, do!
I'm half-crazy, all for the love of you!
It won't be a stylish marriage, I can't afford a carriage
But you'll look sweet upon the seat of a bicycle built for two.

Song 4. "When You Wore a Tulip"

When you wore a tulip, a sweet yellow tulip
And I wore a big red rose
When you caressed me, 'twas then heaven blessed me
What a blessing no one knows
You made life cheery when you called me "dearie"
'Twas down where the blue grass grows
Your lips were sweeter than julep, when you wore a tulip
And I wore a big red rose.

Make every hour sweet as a flower

It's always time to make every hour sweet as a flower. While you are caregiving ask about favorite songs, poems or intimacies that mention flowers.

You might not be the one that has to sing first because people who are dependent on caregivers often enjoy singing and remembering cherished love songs, endearing terms and stories. Actually I find that older men and women often love to sing to us.

I'll never forget the first time I met Gordon at a cardiac rehab in Burlington. I was sent from an agency on aging as his Case Manager to plan his return home. When I walked up to the table where he sat, he launched into a rich vibrato voice serenading me with the grace of a band leader (I found out later he was a performer in the swinging 40s). I had never heard "Out of Nowhere" before and never will again the way Gordon could deliver those vintage jazzy lines:

> "You came to me from out of nowhere.
> You took my heart and found it free
> Wonderful dreams, wonderful schemes out of nowhere,
> Made every hour sweet as a flower to me."

And I did. I schemed to bring him home to his dreams in a trailer park with his wife where he continued serenading us from the bedroom over a microphone voicing the sensuous lyrics of love ballads.

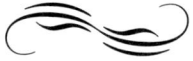

It may sound strange but men (and women) who never sang before often break into songs on their death beds. Recently a dear World War II veteran invited me to his funeral as he sang snatches from "Singing in the Rain" and tossed in and out of sleep on his hospice bed. His daughter told me that he never sang before this, not even in church.

The sound of music and nature is universal. Remember as a caregiver you can make every hour sweet as a flower.

Coaching spirits

Develop a poetry of caregiving…
　　Loving kind words and gestures…
　　　　Reassurances…apologies…
　　　　There, there…I'm sorry you don't feel well today…

Commit yourself to being happy and cheerful…
　　when near the people you are caring for…
　　　　nodding and agreeing…
　　　　　　never arguing, or denying…

Listen every day to people…
　　their dreams, their experiences…
　　　　help…
　　　　　　integrate…
　　　　　　　　their conscious…
　　　　　　　　and unconscious processes…

SIXTEEN
Lullaby memories:
Bewitching tales of the past

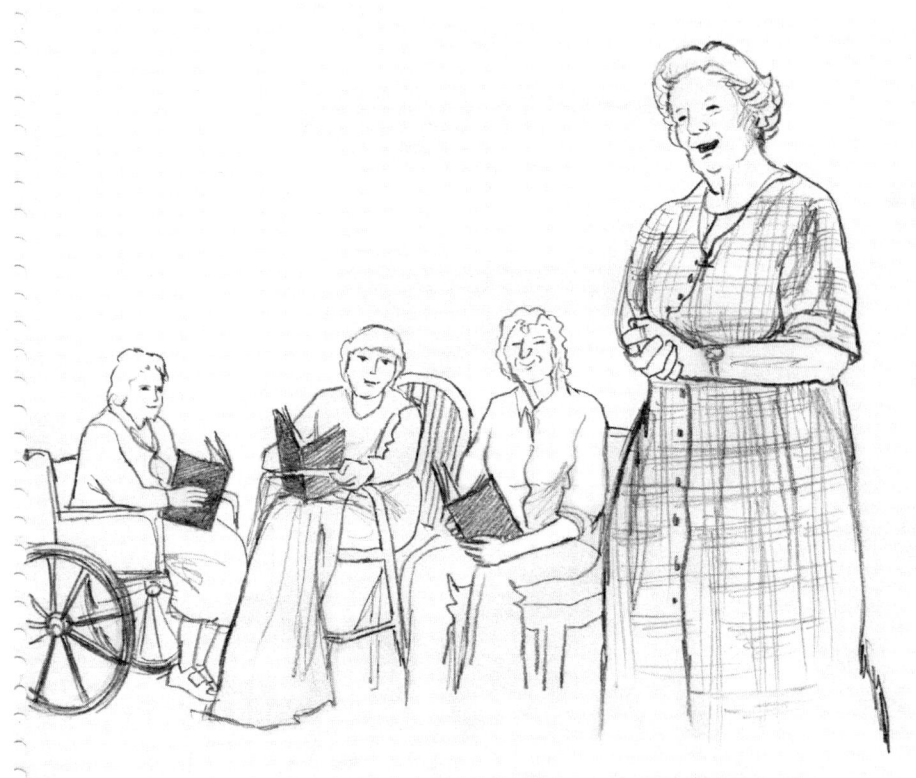

CHELSEA RECITES MANY POEMS FROM MEMORY
while many others wish that they could remember.

A Greek mother

Looking together through colorful photographs of familiar sights provides an opportunity for reminiscence and failure-free activities. Mindful listening to the storytelling soothes the pain and shares the joy.

In Astoria, Maria calls my name out the third story window of yellow brick apartment buildings welcoming me. Her mother Zoe sits at a round table in the parlor with another daughter and granddaughter. Everyone is here to translate.

Zoe chatters Greek and offers me "peps." After a few minutes she comes back from the kitchen broadly grinning. The real treat is candied figs – very sweet green ones in thick syrup from Greece.

Zoe opens the family album and goes through many pictures. Maria protests, "Mama! No!" But then Zoe pulls out a roll of travel posters and begins unrolling them to show me Greece.

It takes all of us to organize these unruly curly posters. Zoe throws them fast as she can as she bends from the waist with her hands and feet deep in the pile. I help Maria catch the posters. We squat to keep them flat. Her other daughter and granddaughter help Zoe who is "cooing" at each scene she unearths and giggling at the crazy papers.

We all sober up when Zoe straightens her back and insists that I take a poster. I refuse at first but quickly catch the commands from Zoe's daughters. "Take one!"

I take a street scene of bright white and blue trimmed sunlit cottages that her granddaughter calls "home."

To this day, the picture helps me recall the day I became one of Zoe's happy Greek daughters in the Greek isles of travel posters.

Leader's Guide: Storytellers

Pictures from family albums, magazines, books, artist's renderings and newspapers are souvenirs of times gone by. Use them to bring back memories and prompt stories.

For this activity, gather and prepare some visual aides.

There are many ways to find the kind of visuals needed for this activity:
- Friends and relatives can provide valuable information: remembered incidents, objects of the past and family photos of childhood, weddings, loved ones, holidays and other significant events.
- Collect art postcards and spread them on the tabletop for elders to pick randomly, muse, sort and tell their own stories.
- Card sets depicting flowers, animals and activities can be found or assembled to stir up memories of pets, favorite things and hobbies such as gardening.
- Even coloring books with their simple outlined images stimulate memories.

    Example: When shown a coloring book picture of a palm tree, a disabled elder from Malta pointed her finger happily at the coconuts. Her eyes lit up with memories of her home island in the Mediterranean Sea.

Begin by showing a picture of a mother or father rocking a baby to sleep in a cradle. Encourage everyone to recall their own experiences putting children to sleep or being put to sleep by their parents. Ask them to recall what they were doing – activities such as sewing, reading a book, whispering to other children – and where they were – for instance, outdoors under trees hearing the sounds of nature.

If you are using personal photos and/or objects of autobiographical meaning, listen to the elder reminiscing and guide the others to listen. Then allow everyone a chance to ask questions.

Assemble photos on a white board or wall so everyone can see the exhibit and share each other's stories.

Exchange these memories with caregivers and staff to pass on information, wisdom and skills that give each person a sense of value and importance of the particular tales of the past however modest the elder's origins.

The first time she felt loved

Childhood reminiscences provide a touchstone for nurturing memories of when we all first knew the security of being loved and cared for.

Betty left Columbia over 60 years ago. After seeing a picture of a horse, she remembered the horses on her father's coffee plantation. She spoke about how strong the horses are in her memories. This triggered her recalling a time when she was a little girl: "My mother was having another baby. My father took me to ride in front of him up high on horseback to my grandmother's house."

Betty straightened her back and leaned forward in her wheelchair. She held her head high as if she still rode horseback with her father. The horse galloped swiftly through a stream. "I held on tight. I could hear my father's heart beating against my body. The next morning when I woke up I asked my grandmother if father really rode me there on horseback. My grandmother said yes he did and that I fell asleep before the end of the ride."

Betty said that this was the first time she knew that her parents really loved her. Because she was one of many children and her parents were very strict with her, Betty said she was not sure of their love until this special ride with her father.

Similarly, objects such as fishing poles, flash lights and aprons are "spirit catchers" and can help elders in their retelling of vital memories.

Mamita, a Puerto Rican grandmother loves to talk about the *"pilon"* used in traditional Puerto Rican cooking:

"When I was a little girl *el pilon* in my house was something special. We used it to press the garlic, all kinds of spices, onions, green pepper, all these herbs that you use to cook. But now you put them in the Osterizer. That's no fun anymore. Now my family criticizes me because I use this. I say I'm proud to use this because this is beautiful, this is natural, this cost me nothing. When I put it on the table, everybody notices, everybody says, Oh, what's that? So then I say very proud, this is from my country. That's a tradition."

Coaching spirits

We all deal with some kind of memory loss. Sometimes we forget things then find them later on. Why do the first fresh violets bring back floods of memories – lavender thoughts of times and loved ones long, long gone? And why does the scent of spring lilacs take our breath away with nostalgia? Are we all adrift on the stream of forgetfulness that the Greeks called the River Lethe?

Flowers and horses, these universal images stir memories that are still there on the Alzheimer's journey. While living in a remote village on the Aleutian islands, I had the opportunity to witness horses roaming freely in and out of town. This rhythmic poem may help your country partners remember the beauty of horses.

One by one the horses come up the beach from town:
one white, a chestnut, and a paint, led by two velvety browns.

Here and there they stop to dig, to sift the morning snow.
Like drifting ghosts they softly flee before the sleepy children know.

To fields beyond the town they go
where sun can reach them, quiet, slow.

The white one sits like a guardian sphinx
to watch the sun fill wakening streets.

Later children quietly follow, two or three at a time
to offer timid grabs of grasses to the nocturnal ghosts of town.

One by one the horses come up the beach from town:
one white, a chestnut, and a paint, led by two velvety browns.

SEVENTEEN
Sing the blues: Bonding with cries

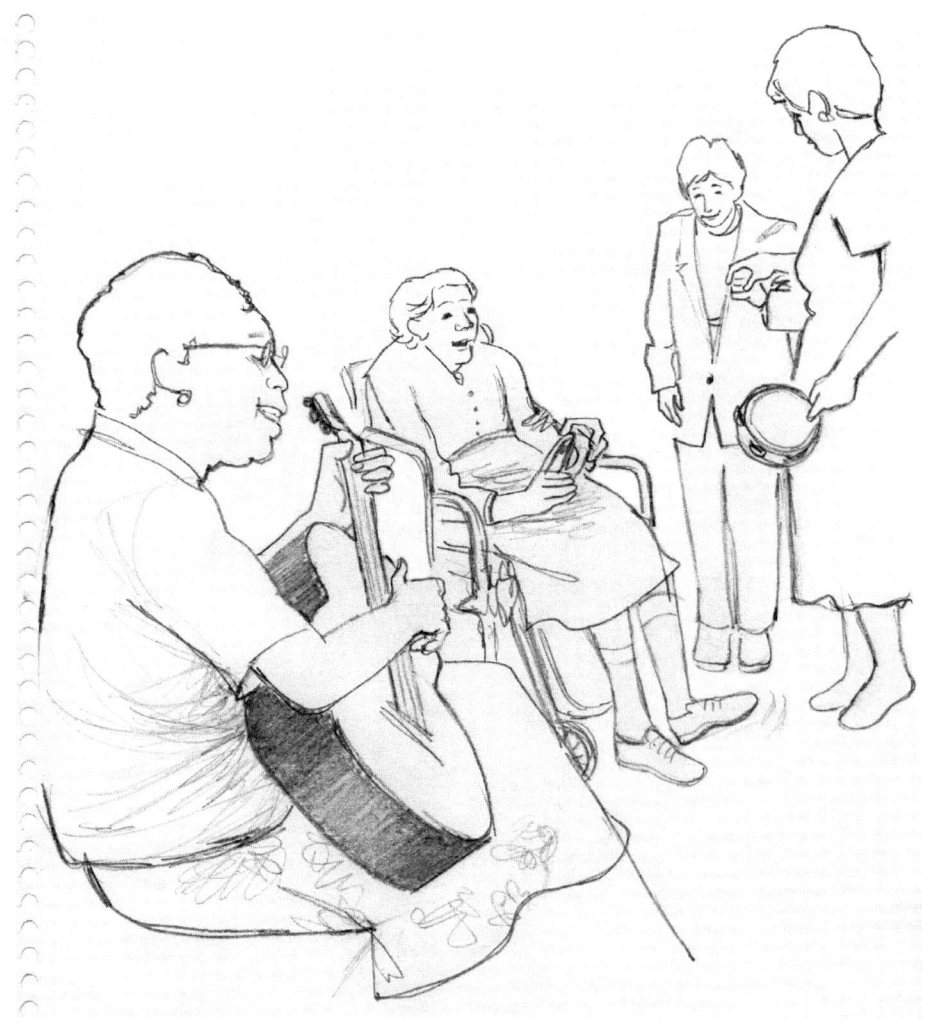

ELLEN WALKS
while they all sing "Peg of My Heart."

In the beginning, there was the blues

In difficult times – storms, wars, separations, losses – people soothe their children and others by taking time to talk, listen, sing, reminisce and tell stories.

A mother and daughter in Manhattan's East Village cry a lot at bedtime because daddy is no longer living at home. They sing – "My Bonnie lies over the ocean, My Bonnie lies over the sea, My Bonnie lies over the ocean, Oh bring back my Bonnie to me."

In Brooklyn's Bay Ridge, a Danish-American grandmother sings "*Sov, mit barn, sov laenge*" (Sleep my child, sleep a long time), a lullaby everybody in Denmark knows. The mother is trying to make her child comfortable by telling her not to worry. She brushes away the flies as she confides her true feelings in these words translated from the Danish poem by Christian Richardt:

> Vigorous as wine
> You grow in my mind,
> Grow out of the arms of your mother
> Into the dangers of the world.
> Red roses of happiness
> Glow only between thorns.
> The thorn is for me
> While I save the rose for you.

Leader's Guide: Memorials that evoke emotions

Set aside a time for a remembrance service every few months or so. You can invite a member of the clergy or local hospice bereavement staff to help present a special program. A poignant memory of someone, a reading for example "My carnation," can set the tone. Sensory items help create positive emotional memories. Give a fresh flower to each person in memory of a lost loved one.

The staff wants to share memories of recent losses. People with dementia summon up just as much emotion remembering mothers, fathers, brothers, sisters and spouses from long, long ago.

"Bring Back My Bonnie" expresses the loss and longing for a beloved hero to return home. Those whom we care for are often experiencing a similar painful longing for lost loves and past dreams. Repetitive words and melody encourage people to participate in singing and moving their bodies.

Sitting in a circle holding hands if possible, sing the chorus a few times.

Leader directs and models:
Start with the chorus and sway in one direction on "bring" and the other direction on "back."

Bring back, bring back
Oh bring back my Bonnie to me, to me
Bring back, bring back
Oh, bring back my Bonnie to me

My Bonnie lies over the ocean
My Bonnie lies over the sea
My Bonnie lies over the ocean
Oh, bring back my Bonnie to me

Oh blow ye winds over the ocean
And blow ye winds over the sea
Oh blow ye winds over the ocean
And bring back my Bonnie to me

The winds have blown over the ocean
The winds have blown over the sea
The winds have blown over the ocean
And brought back my Bonnie to me

Ask participants to say the name of the person, pet, place or thing that they want to remember. Then, singing the chorus together, replace the name "Bonnie."

Example:
Leader: Mary, tell us the name of someone you want to remember today.
Mary answers: Maria.
Leader: We can sing "Bring back my Maria to me."

Everyone together sings:

Bring back, bring back
Oh bring back my Maria to me.
Bring back, bring back
Oh, bring back my Maria to me

Honoring diversity

Many therapists note that our older adults with dementia are more there than most people will admit. They are like mystics out in spiritual realms. Now and then, if we caregivers listen well enough to the person's experiences, we will be rewarded with sage communications from them.

Take Lucas for example: Before coming into the nursing home, Lucas was a farmer. In his 80's now he usually sits alone in his room. As if in a cave near darkness, he prefers not to put on a light or attend programs. He is a friend of the shadows and bird songs.

In early spring, I take Lucas outside to the gazebo. He likes listening to the birds and remembers something from long ago. In a voice soft and slow, he speaks:

"See, See, See.
Where? Where? Where?
Here. Here. Here.
Oh see me! Oh see me! Oh see me!"

Listening to Lucas' rhythmic sound memory reminds me of the baby starling that came out of the bushes where it had escaped after I chased the cat away. The baby bird nodded its head side to side; again it hopped then stopped to screech then remain quiet and still. This went on for awhile. I could not hear or see what the little bird was sensing. Still I listened to the bird's reality. At this point, I saw the mother bird flitting through low branches at the end of the yard calling her baby to her. Next the lost bird hopped quickly through the grass to the trees where mother waited.

Coaching spirits

Sometimes it takes very little to brighten-up the day like in this memory of bringing my mother a very small violet bouquet.

Blue spotted sky
Over red spotted fields
Violet bouquets
In the red maple April spring
Eastside Albia

Coming down to Plum Avenue
Carrying 7 violets
Amethyst butterflies
Between my thumb and forefinger
Baby blue baby violets
faces short-stemmed.
"Take care of them, here mother."

She says, "How they're so beautiful.
How they take care of themselves out there."
We float them in a shot glass
in front of a recent family bride.

I gave her seven baby violets
And realized she is always wearing
a light violet dress.

EIGHTEEN
Following traditions: Positive feelings of old sheets and vintage tunes

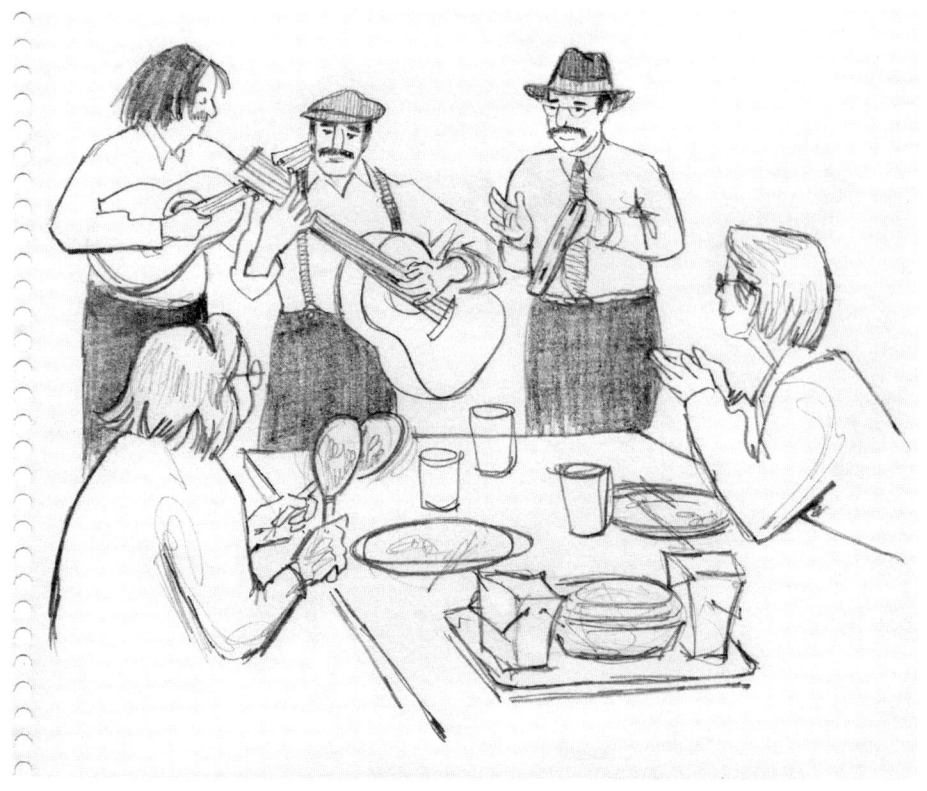

"EN MI VIEGO SAN JUAN"
fills the kitchen with nostalgic memories of old San Juan.

Sounds and smells that soothe

A children's day care director talked about the importance of rest periods. He explained that the positive feelings associated with the smell of the time and place where the child falls asleep at home helps the child to relax and rest in the day care center. He made a point, "I tell the parents to bring in the old sheets, not new ones."

The day care center director got into telling us what puts him to sleep on Sunday afternoons – the sound of wind in leaves, a familiar smell, the low murmurs of people in another room talking.

This director insists that kids need the rest: "They are pushed all day in our culture. Some will not allow themselves to fall asleep." So he employs techniques that do the trick. He makes soothing sounds. Using a pan of water, he splashes it like waves over and over. As evidence of its effectiveness, children ask for this.

Leader's Guide: Harvest sensory treasures

Look for the traditions, music and songs of cultural identity. These customs are often known by an entire community that shares a common ground of heritage, birthplace, childhood, workplace, religion and language.

Nature gives us many cues that reduce stress. It is reported that most people imagine themselves outdoors in natural settings when they are trying to calm down. We work in healthcare industries and cannot get outside to natural panaceas enough. What can we do to care more for ourselves and others in interior environments?

Bring seasonal offerings to men and women. There is no end to the rhythmic treasures we can harvest. Often these surprises are free for the taking – springtime pussy willows, golden forsythia, purple violets, pink apple blossoms, mint leaves, lilacs, strawberries, apples, autumn leaves, bright orange pumpkins for carving.

Stanley's beloved wife passed away a year ago. This first spring as a widower he gave out bundles of rhubarb to people who would promise to bake a strawberry rhubarb pie and give him a piece in memory of his dear wife who made the best pies ever. He praised the widow who sat next to him at support group. "She made a five-star pie!" he said and smiled thankfully as he put his arm around her for a moment and patted her shoulder.

Even those who are on restricted diets can enjoy summertime corn on the cob. Shuck it together – touch the cool yellow kernels and slippery silk.

This practice helps maintain cultural roots and identity throughout life. Keep track of familiar and favorite sensory experiences so that appropriate interventions can be offered when needed.

Herbalist Colleen K. Dodt is the author of *The Essential Oils Book*. In a section entitled "Caring for the elderly and sick," Dodt suggests peeling a fresh orange beside the bedside of an ailing elder or sprinkling rosemary essential oil on a hair brush and enjoying your elder's response to an aromatic hair brushing. Dodt writes about doing all these things when she was acting as guardian to a woman in a nursing home: "Mildred's whole sense of being would change after these times together. I know the quality of her stay was greatly enhanced by the use of pure essential oils in her room."

"I also think the nurses were so attentive in part, because of how comfortable her room felt with its sweetly scented contents." Not only will your elders sense of being change when sensory experiences are heightened, but also the quality of care given will be enhanced, herbalist Dodt testifies.

Or invent your own traditions.

There is a storehouse of associations available once you pick a unifying theme. I collaborated with residents in a retirement community on several invigorating and original celebration days. Their religious order already had daylong theme days when everyone participated. The King's Day tradition began early in January when a bean cake was served. Whoever got the piece of cake with a black bean in it became the king for a day. Not only did the lucky overnight royalty get to choose a queen for the day but also the theme for the King's Day that generated all activities, foods served, movies and other entertainments.

One king picked *The King and I* as the theme. We re-created the march of the Siamese children. The king and queen entered the community room hand-in-hand and doffed their crowns throwing gold foil-wrapped chocolate coins to their lowly subjects. Carolyn, a talented retired music teacher, gave a memorable program called "Name That Tune." She played the first few notes of each unforgettable tune from the movie on the piano and audience members had to guess which song it was. Then we all joined in, singing along.

Another year the king wanted a Spanish theme. Included on that day were a mouth-watering flan, a traveling trio with guitars and hand drums who wandered the dining hall and hallways visiting many room-bound elders, serenading everyone. "En Mi Viejo San Juan" filled the day with echoes of "adios" in old San Juan. English and Spanish versions of the movie *The Milagro Beanfield War* were shown simultaneously in two different recreation rooms. We broke out all the maracas, shakers – and other instruments and we jammed and danced with our visiting trio. King's Day filled the winter months with joyful expectations, limitless creativity and precious memories preserved in pictures taken of the merry moments.

Another series of special days emerged from a collaboration with a resident who practiced massage and aromatherapy. This talented therapist with an equally talented staff produced days designed to celebrate and educate everyone about the uses of natural essential oils to lift the spirits and enhance relaxation, provoke feelings and memories.

Flyers were distributed to advertise the theme of the day with requests that everyone including all staff wear the color of the essential oil and be ready to contribute stories and memories associated with the fragrance. Themes included Orange Day, Lemon Day, Lavender Day, Ginger Day and Rose Day. Evergreen Day was especially appropriate on the New Year with pine scent to clear the mind and clean the environment.

Activities, some outrageous, all fun were:
- Everyone got pinned with the color, often just a simple ribbon bow for the day
- A lecture with demonstrations about the therapeutic properties of the oil
- Electric diffusers gently emitted whiffs of the elixir in a common room all day
- Prizes like sachets, cleaners, teas and foods were given
- Dramas were presented (Ginger Day included gingerbread houses and an enactment of a scene from *Hansel and Gretel*).

Herbalist and author Dodt adds that "The association between freshly laundered clothes and lavenders dates back centuries when bed linens were hung upon lavender hedges to dry in the sun." So exploring using aromatherapy and natural remedies can evoke deep and sage results in the growing aging community of diverse backgrounds and cultures.

Gershwin tunes

When I booked a popular jazz duet to do a holiday music program I wasn't sure of the appropriateness of my choice. The audience was a group of retired nuns. Several of the women had been music teachers. Many came from families where the piano was the central focus at home in the early 1900s.

After a prayer service the Sisters – ranging in age from 60 to 100, some in wheelchairs and others with walkers – clustered around the food offerings and chatted. In the connecting parlor, the singer scatted microphone checks in front of her music stand draped with a sequined scarf.

I tipped off the musicians about the audience's interest in the words and music of Ira and George Gershwin. Drawn into the piano parlor by the improvisations, the Sisters seated themselves and I introduced the musicians. The vocalist's opening song lines, "Picture me upon your knee, tea for two and two for tea," bubbled over with lovers' lyrics. I looked around at her attentive audience surprised to see that they were mouthing these spicy lyrics about lovers!

Love resonated through the audience during an intimate rendition of "Our Love Is Here to Stay." Everyone sang together at the end:

> "In time the Rockies may crumble,
> Gibraltar may tumble,
> They're only made of clay,
> But our love is here to stay."

Refreshed faces beamed with joyful recall of the old favorite romantic love songs.

Coaching spirits

Assist the recall of favorite songs or music,
    events and issues…
        that arise along with the music.

Ask where…
    When…
        and why…
        the song was being listened to,
        played or sung.

Encourage the singing of the song
        and the recall of the words,
        and repeat references to these songs in future music sessions.

For those who are less able,
the music experience can be done solo,
without a leader,
while listening to recorded or live music.

Participants may sing inwardly to themselves,
    perhaps only lip-syncing now and then
    between seemingly aimless but therapeutic movements and moods.
        The experience of being alone with palliative music allows
        release of deep tensions and access to inner harmony.

NINETEEN
Power songs and prayers:
The soulful opportunities of traditions

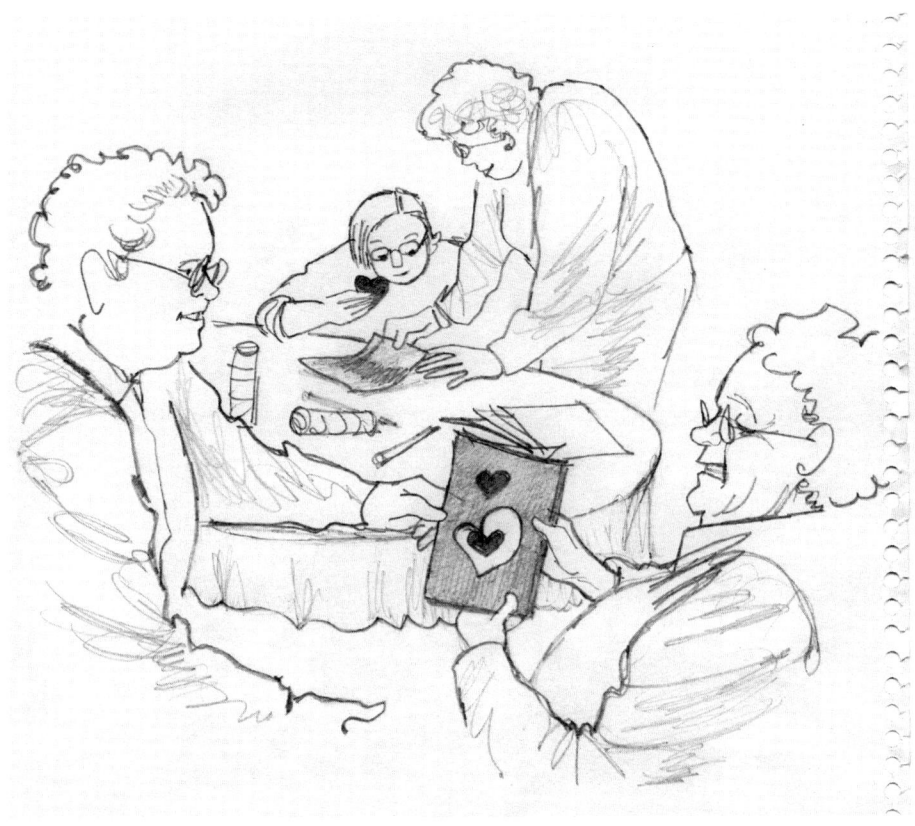

VALENTINE'S DAY
A day of the heart shared by everyone.

Nurturing moonlit memories

When I was collecting lullabies in New York City I found that "Silent Night" was sung all year round often due to lack of other repertory. There is song poverty because songs and singing are often not passed on. I named my organization "Song Bank" with the goal of collecting and sharing these songs like treasures.

Ruth Crawford Seeger suggested this idea in *American Folk Songs for Children*: "Many of us open a savings account at the bank when a child is born, and add layer after layer of small deposits which he can later draw on for a college education," she wrote in the book's introduction. "Perhaps a fund of songs might be begun as early, and added to layer after layer – an ever-growing wealth of materials which he can draw on at will and can take along with him as links from himself to the various aspects of the culture he will be going out to meet."

Marisa, a school teacher in New York City, suddenly remembered with deep emotion the poem that her sweet and loving mom used to recite to her at her bedside when she was very young in the Philippines. When Marisa went to pre-school, she learned it as a song. Marisa translated:

> Dear little moon
> High over head
> Shines gently down
> On my small white bed.

Marisa added with a yearning tremble in her voice – "I was walking home the other night in Brooklyn and I saw the moon."

"Beautiful memories of the past flooded my mind," she sighed.

A haunting moonlight shone out her dark eyes as she looked lovingly homeward.

Leader's Guide: Simple songs

Have you ever wondered why a person with memory loss can sing all the words to a Christmas song but not be able to respond to a simple question or remember how to take a step or use a spoon?

Here are some songs and rhymes that can be a source of encouragement and connection. The activities recall the simple affirming words and tunes we may have learned as children that still have power to awaken hope and faith.

Nursery rhymes

Begin by gathering all the stuffed animals in the room. Review Mother Goose Nursery Rhymes for animal references. For example:

> Three Little Kittens, they lost their mittens
> And they began to cry,
> "Oh mother dear we greatly fear,
> That we have lost our mittens."
> "What! Lost your mittens, you naughty kittens
> Then you shall have no pie!
> Mee-ow, Mee-ow, Mee-ow, Mee-ow
> Then you shall have no pie."

Gather around the table, and one by one introduce the stuffed animals, in any order (size, color, species). Name them, give sensory directions (soft, shiny, sweet, pink) and make a game of giving everyone a pet for the day. Then go ahead and play.

Use springboards of babble. Meows and quacks can lead into a delightful dance of conversation. Even few discernable words evoke feelings such as - shrieks of delight, fountains of laughter, playful mock dramas.

"Hush Little Baby"

This activity challenges participants to think of rhyming words to complete the song

A song such as "Hush Little Baby" has a game inside. You have to use the word in one sentence to make up a second sentence.

Here is the most common version of this old folksong. Have fun singing by waiting for someone to fill in the end rhyme of each couplet. Accept all variations, even non-rhyming words so you can get to the end of the song each time you sing it together.

Anything goes.

> Hush little baby, don't say a word,
> Papa's gonna buy you a mocking bird.
>
> If that mocking bird doesn't sing,
> Papa's gonna buy you a diamond ring.
>
> If that diamond ring turns brass,
> Papa's gonna buy you a looking glass.
>
> If that looking glass gets broke,
> Papa's gonna buy you a billygoat.
>
> If that billygoat won't pull,
> Papa's gonna buy you a cart and bull.
>
> If that cart and bull turn over,
> Papa's gonna buy you a dog named Rover.
>
> If that dog named Rover won't bark,
> Papa's gonna buy you a horse and cart.
>
> If that horse and cart fall down,
> You'll still be the sweetest little baby in town.

"Kumbaya"

Ask if anyone knows what the word "kumbaya" means. "Kumbaya" is dialect (African Angolan) for "Come by here."

Start with the chorus:

> Kumbaya, my Lord, kumbaya
> Kumbaya, my Lord, kumbaya
> Kumbaya, my Lord, kumbaya
>
> O Lord, kumbaya
>
> Someone's laughing, Lord, kumbaya
> Someone's laughing, Lord, kumbaya
> Someone's laughing, Lord, kumbaya
>
> O Lord, kumbaya

Variations:

> Someone's crying, Lord, kumbaya
> Someone's praying, Lord, kumbaya
> Someone's singing, Lord, kumbaya

You can extend this song endlessly by singing each other's names instead of "someone" and introducing new action words instead of "sleeping." Example:

> Rosemarie's smiling, my Lord, kumbaya
> Rosemarie's smiling, my Lord, kumbaya
> Rosemarie's smiling, my Lord, kumbaya
>
> O Lord, kumbaya

Variation:

> Eddie's laughing, Lord…

"Starlight, Star Bright"

This is another example of the power of songs, chants, prayers, and words in our daily lives. We probably all know "Starlight, Star Bright." It's a nursery rhyme that contains a simple charm.

Read or sing "Starlight, Star Bright," and then prompt memories of learning this nursery rhyme.

> Starlight, star bright,
> The first star I see tonight,
> I wish I may, I wish I might,
> Have the wish I wish tonight.

Ask:

"Do you remember what you saw out your window at night as a child? Tell us about it."

"What did you wish for as a child?"

"What do you wish for now?"

"What do you think the stars see and hear when they look down on us?"

Sharing prayers

Many people teach their children to pray before going to bed. A prayer is often said repeatedly, sometimes all your life.

Ask those in your care if they learned this as a childhood prayer:

> Now I lay me down to sleep
> I pray the Lord my soul to keep
> If I should die before I wake,
> I pray the Lord my soul to take.

Discuss feelings about this prayer, leading into any fears that your participants may remember or have now about falling asleep at night.

Ask:

"Did you say a special prayer at night as a child?"

"Where did you say it? Were you alone?"

"Did anyone pray aloud with you, and teach you your prayers?"

"What was that prayer?"

"Do you say a prayer at night now?"

"Who do you want to pray for now?"

"What are the words of your prayer?"

Sundowning

"Sundowning" is the term used to describe the agitation that occurs regularly in the afternoon for some people with dementia. This agitation is thought to be a chemical reaction in the brain that is triggered by the waning light at the end of the day.

Megan's Irish father was a singer. She remembers his voice whenever we play Irish sing-alongs although she refuses to sing a note. But his music can calm down Megan at the end of the day when she is sundowning.

After the five o'clock supper, Megan's agitation and anxiety often increase. She wheels her chair up the hall looking for a way to the elevator, the next floor, Chicago and home. While I work in my office, I play "The Three Irish Tenors in Belfast" video for Megan in the activities room across the hall. Forgetting her fear for a moment, she reaches for tablecloths to fold and pulls a straw hat out of the prop box, playfully putting it on her head. Between songs, Megan looks up and comments, "My father stopped singing."

I soothe Megan by saying that her father needs to rest his voice now. I invite her to go back down the hall to her room. As we approach the nurse calls, "I like your hat, Megan!" She gracefully accepts the compliment and calmly adjusts to sitting with others waiting in the community room for her turn to go to bed.

Regularly scheduled late afternoon activities can also address frustration and boredom, behaviors that are similar to sundowning. Often I have a music program at four o'clock before supper. I walk with the elders like a tireless mother at the end of day. This is a wonderful rhythm for each of us to get into while listening to gentle music and singing along.

Ellen, the author of many books, never recovered from a catastrophic illness. She usually sits smiling through the first half of the music and movement program. Then she reaches for me and, beaming a very wide-open grin, she pulls herself up from her chair and begins to walk in rhythm with me. I put one arm around her back as we begin to dance. The music carries us easily like summer breezes. We sing along as we step, stopping to visit each person in the circle.

Laura, a retired librarian in her late eighties, shakes the maraca and greets Ellen with smiles, cheerfully calling "Congratulations!"

Ann shakes the tambourine toward Ellen, and Ellen communicates with another beautiful smile. Virginia rings the bells for Ellen who smiles to her greeting. We walk in dance rhythms back and forth. Ellen takes my hand and gently turns to the other end of the hall. This continues perhaps 10 to 12 minutes until trays arrive.

Then Ellen greets the nurses with the wonderful warm and glowing smile and sits down to eat supper.

Coaching spirits

Caregivers' Promise

As long as
>You live,
>I am your
>Best caregiver

>The bondage
>Creates the need to
>Sing and dance
>Together
>To relate
>To lighten up
>The load

>>Sing
>>As you
>>Dance
>>Your caregiving

>>>Dance
>>>As long as they live and breathe
>>>Laughing
>>>As long as you care
>>>Caring while letting go.

TWENTY
Finding home in lullabies:
The longing for someone somewhere

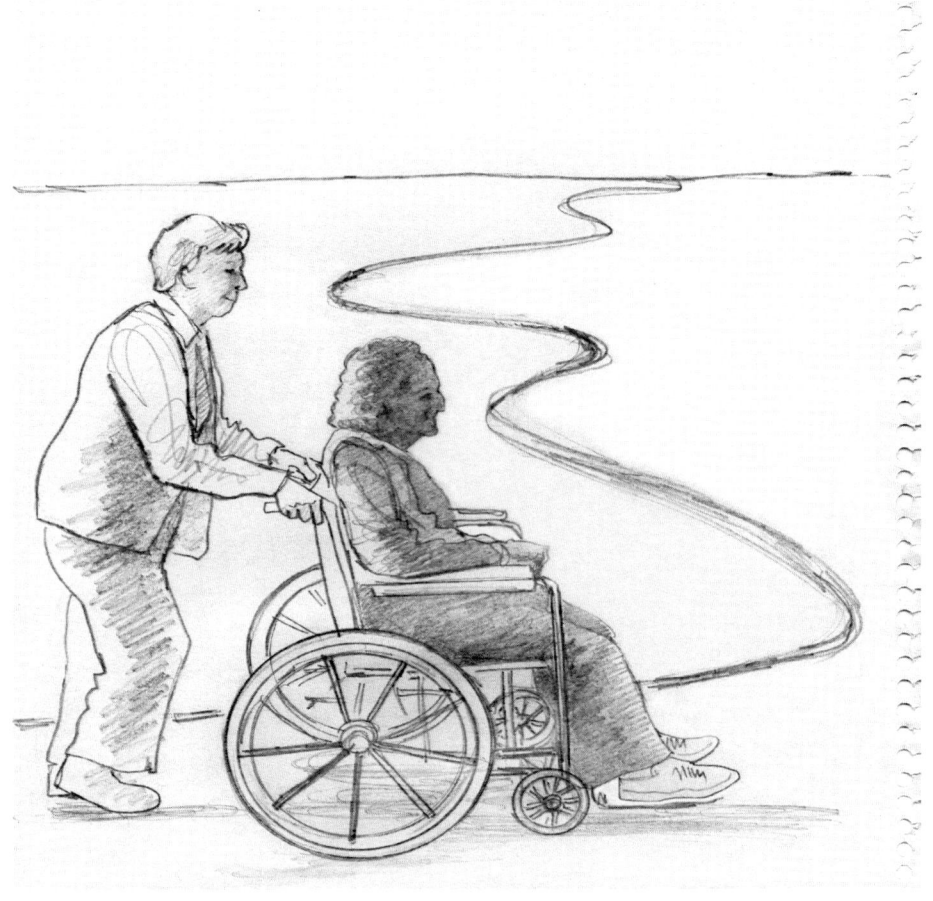

THE UNKNOWN
becomes known with compassion.

In the beginning, there was mother and home

> "Singing to soothe one's self is seen in children's stories where lost children sing to themselves while wandering in the woods as a means of dispelling their fear."
>
> From Christine Knowles reflections on *As Long as You Sing, I'll Dance*

Home is never forgotten. As transitions are made, people find a new home, or make a home. Our elders often have to share their home. They say even when they are in the nursing home they have to go "home" always remembering the first home where they were safe, intimately held, protected, connected to their mothers' heartbeats. Mother and home means being loved and nurtured, feeling positive, peaceful and safe.

A 10-year old who was orphaned by the April 1991 cyclone in Bangledesh was quoted in a national news story as saying: "I was terrified. So I sang lullabies." When hospitalized soldiers after World War II needed special treatment for trauma, physicians sought out their mothers' lullabies. These tragic stories attest to the power of lullabies to soothe, relax and reassure – no matter the circumstances.

People remember lullabies long after they forget the languages of ancestors. In lullabies persist forms, codes and secrets of the past that soothe and relax. The lullaby carries keys that open windows on identity. Any song that expresses the longing for home can become a lullaby. For example, Van Morrison's "Into the Mystic": "…And when the fog horn blows I will be coming home…. I want to rock your gypsy soul just like way back in the days of old and together we will float into the mystic."

Relaxation techniques make use of the power of the voice to lead the imagination to quiet spaces. The voice then guides us to see, hear and feel comfortable thereby relaxing the conscious mind so the body can fall asleep.

African mothers keep their very young children closely wrapped. Many women carry babies on their backs. One Nigerian mother explained: "To put the baby to sleep, you walk around. You stamp your feet and shake your body. As if you are dancing, the way you dance to rock and roll music here in the States. You carry this baby and while you are doing that, you sing and shake your body up and down. Then the baby gets the feeling of rocking and that keeps him quiet. It's the totality of the whole thing – the rhythm of the song with the rhythm of the body. The child stops crying, feels warm. Even if you are not carrying the child, laying the child down on a bed, chair or the floor on the wrappers works. You clap your hands. The child feels your clapping and smells his mother's scent on the wrapper nearby. This puts the child to sleep."

Leader's Guide: Going home

Listening and Quiet Activity

Blow bubbles together while listening to "Over the Rainbow" (the original version by Judy Garland, if you can get it) or find another recording that you think is a touchstone for the people you care for. Listen to the music with a quiet meditative activity like bubble blowing, drawing, coloring or painting, stretching or body movements.

Take a childhood walk home

As the leader, do whatever is possible to make the room a relaxing therapeutic space. Lower the lights, use soft music, and most importantly, find your own calm, quiet breath and loving attitude. Make sure people are comfortable.

Explain that you are all going on a memory journey, together, but everyone will go to his or her own past. Because they will be following your voice, be sure not to rush your sentences and pause often for brief silences. Breathe deeply.

Leader: "Close your eyes and become aware of your breathing for a moment."

(Pause for a few moments.)

"Now picture yourself on the way home from school with Mommy or your older brother or whoever safely brought you home." (Pause again)

"See yourself scurrying ahead."

"Now gradually in your mind's eye, picture yourself throwing your leg over a fence and climbing into a little park on the way home." (Pause again)

"Very slowly, you roll in the long cool grass. Feel this happening as you do it. Feel all the grass you have to yourself. Smell the grass…smell the earth… press your whole stomach into it and breathe deeply. Feel the sun on your back and the little blades of grass against your face."

(Pause for a few moments.)

"Take off your shoes and wiggle your toes in the grass. Now notice the wildflowers or dandelions or something else you see there in the little park that you want to take home with you. Go ahead and pick it up."

"Look up at the sky… the clouds… the sun." (Pause)

"Then, as you hear your name called, you climb over the fence and meet your Mommy or your brother to go home again." (Pause)

"Now open your eyes slowly, and come back to the room."

Talk about this activity.

At the end of imagining a childhood walk home from school, Carol continued the story. Everyone's eyes were wide open as she started to describe in detail her little park and the bird she wanted to take home with her. Ann told us about a man who had entered into her imaginary journey. She told him to leave because it was her peaceful place. Roddy said that after listening to their descriptive stories and breathing in and out he felt very relaxed.

"Home, Home on the Range"

Our guest musician and Rabbi called his January program of prayer and song, "Bringing in the New Year." When he opened with – of all the wild choices – a cowboy serenade, our grinning minstrel explained he was trying to expand his range of songs beyond his own Hebrew and Yiddish culture. The Rabbi thought this would be a good opener for the New Year.

Guitar slung over his dark suit jacket he hollered, "Home, home on the range." Rabbi wears the traditional *yarmulke* (not a cowboy hat) as he sings. The white-haired men and women in the Community Room were transfixed. They joined in the wacky chorus with wild abandon each time the rabbi came to "Home, home on the range…"

Feeling at home in this American song, they cheered the Rabbi for his unusual opening song. They repeated to each other "Home…where the deer and the antelope play…." "Home, where seldom is heard a discouraging word and the skies are not cloudy all day."

Sometimes the context of an old rag, in this case a 19th century traditional American cowboy song, makes a song fresh and powerful as the national anthem.

The Rabbi touched our deeper feelings that winter day. The simple lyrics of a joyful easier time became a deeply bonding and healing spiritual experience.

Finding home in "Home, Home on the Range" helped us practice the harmony, safety, joy and togetherness of being at home any time, any place.

Coaching spirits

My mother loved to watch the birds and the flowers. I write poems about the birds and flowers to find my attachment with her again.

The truth is I never was able to care for her in her last years of battling Alzheimer's disease and aging. I am healing this loss of my ability to care for her with musical poetic images affirming our best times together. She is my goddess and muse of nurturing natural powers.

How like a woman
She bends
The robin over the nest's edge
Tucking each straw into its place
Cupping the weave
With the rounds of her shape
How like my mother
She bends
The robin over the nest's edge.

CODA
The "bye-bye" in lullabies
Peaceful ways to make clear closures

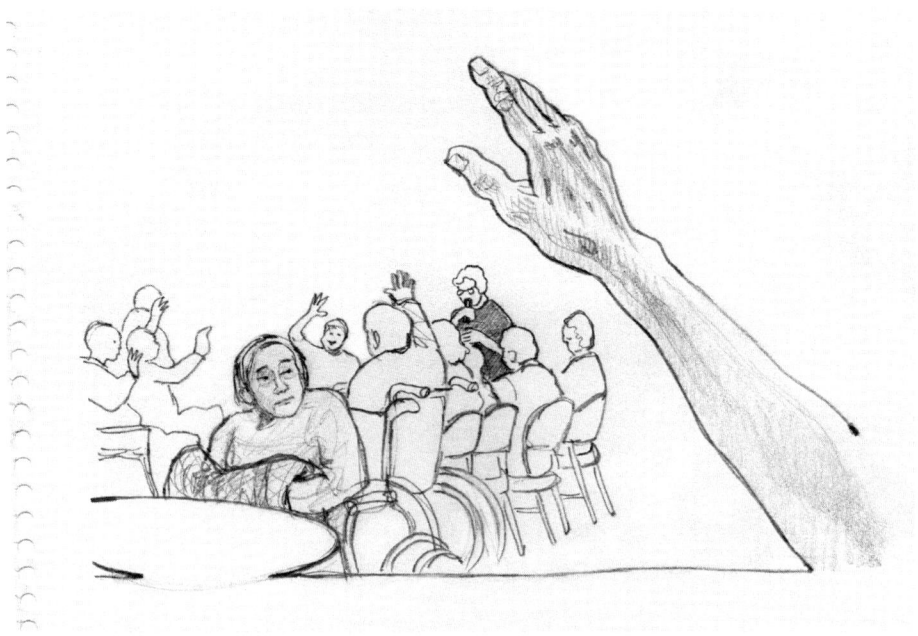

A PEACEFUL UNDERSTANDING
of our transitions is a benediction beyond words.

> In the Middle Ages the word "lull-a-by" was used as a peaceful farewell.
>
> You can say "lullaby" instead of good-bye. Lullaby means good-bye.

I see in the springtime luxuriant irises blooming. Again, I will have to let them go to the wind and the changeful weather reciting the words of an old haiku I wrote to some invisible presence years ago: *So many irises / Go home silently with you / Surrendering perfume.*

I have dealt with my own transience while writing poems that help me stay in the present moment. As I recorded lullabies in New York City, I experienced some of the most moving experiences of the transitional use of songs – the soothing tone of the unmediated voices; the improvisational scat-like echo between bodies accompanied by the images of poetry.

We often experience caregiving while letting go. So we must find peaceful ways to let a person know what's happening and make clear closures. Music is a blessing to be offered. Music guides people of all ages. Just as the worldwide traditions of lullabies have developed to help people in all cultures say goodbye for awhile, music is a guide to be offered as part of palliative care at the last hours of a person's life.

When Doris returned from the hospital, she was no longer eating and her lungs were deeply congested. I greeted her, identifying myself by first name. She roused, repeating my name fondly.

"You were very sick, Doris," I tried to comfort her, bending over her bed and stroking her forehead gently. She was the rhythm keeper of our music sessions. She found and kept the beat of every tune accompanying live piano, recorded music or sing-a-longs on the two-note rhythm sticks or bells.

Now I smiled seeing her lying in bed still tapping one foot underneath the sheet keeping rhythm with her soul. "Would you like some music?"

She responded a muted "Yes!"

"What kind of music would you like, Doris?"

In a heartbeat she answered, "Benediction."

Hispanic children tell me they ask their parents to give them a blessing at night. The child asks, "*Mama, bendicion?*" Their mother replies, *"Que dios te bendigas"* ("God bless you, my child"). This means she is asking God to give her child his blessing too. I also say good-bye long distance to my husband's Puerto Rican family the same way, asking for *"bendicion."*

When caregivers and families find a way to communicate together that enriches both giver and receiver, there is peace in the house. A peaceful understanding of our transitions is a benediction beyond words.

I included lullabies and poetry as farewells for both my mother and father. These words are from "Eulogy for Marcella Mae Gontier Lebentritt, December 30, 1988."

> When I think of my mother,
> I think of a double rainbow over Dyken Pond
> And the song, "Somewhere over the rainbow,
> Way up high, there's a land
> That I heard of once in a lullaby."
> When I think of my mom,
> I remember being held in her arms.
> My mother passed on the act of mothering to me.
> The mother rests too. She rests in the child's rest.
> "Rest is a communion of love" between us.
> I want to give my mother rest now.
> "Bye-bye, Marcella."
> We love you.

Though shadows dark
Fall on your bed of bark
Have no fear
For mother is near
Mn – Mn – Mn – Mn

From *Lullabies of the World* (1967)
Dorothy Berliner Commins, comp.
From Queensland, Australia

Acknowledgements

When I received the first grant for "New York City Lullabies" in 1981, a colleague remarked prophetically that I was beginning a life work. So now decades later I am not surprised to see this book exists as a memoir as well as a resource for caregivers.

My mother and father devoted their lives with patience and support as I vacillated between a career in healthcare, marriage, education and the creative arts. It was a bumpy road but I hope this book amounts to something they can see with pride from their celestial guardian thrones above me.

I want to acknowledge and thank the hundreds of adults and children in New York City who allowed me to come into their lives, sometimes homes, sometimes bedrooms and beds, to record and share their lullaby traditions. It is the voice of the people that carries on the traditions that bring peace in this troubled world. Without the professional guidance and collaboration of independent producer Karen Pearlman and consultant Dr. Barbara Kirshenblatt-Gimblett, founder of the Performing Arts Program at New York University, my lullaby work would never have emerged internationally.

This manuscript began when professional writer Karen Kernan, also a friend and collaborator on the lullaby project, encouraged me to collect my lullaby-based activities for caregivers of the elderly and terminally ill. Karen provided some of the original templates for the design of this book. She also served as an editor in the first drafts of the work. Author Meisha Rosenberg, my neighbor and friend, also assisted me with her precise editorial reviews of earlier drafts.

Melissa Mykal Batalin at the The Troy Book Makers patiently guided me through several years of refining my work. She referred me to a city desk editor at the Albany *Times Union*. It was Rob Brill who "brilled" this manuscript with his enthusiastic brilliance. It was Rob who (like the Robin Hood of old) shot the arrows into my consciousness. He said that I had to put myself into the book: Julia Lebentritt, a lullaby collector in New York City; Julia, a caregiver, Director of Activities and Bereavement Facilitator; Julia, also known as Leben, a poet and M.F.A. in Creative Writing; and finally Julia, the only *Lullabologist* on Earth who wants to speak to the world about the need for lullabies in the world.

January 2011, I met artist Jeanne Benas at a workshop for writers (again in my own backyard) at The Troy Book Makers. Almost all of Jeanne's pencil sketches portray scenes/images gathered from photographs from my lullaby project in New York City and my caregiving activities at Kenwood. Jeanne and I decided that we liked the pencil sketches rather than making final ink illustrations for a special reason: the medium is the message here – Jeanne's illustrations are spontaneous and fresh as if the artist is drawing live models on site. This suggests that artistic caregivers and/or seniors/clients/patients may also enjoy drawing or photographing their daily activities for future displays and documentation of their lives.

Jeanne Benas' creative abilities contribute to my work as a multicultural tool for diverse populations and intergenerational causes. I am very grateful to her for interpreting the diversity of the gestures that articulate my communication concepts with joy, warmth and most of all good humor. Don't miss the irony in some of her takes on the caregiver and the "audience members."

There are numerous other colleagues, family and friends to thank along this lullaby journey. I have asked Armando Soto millions of time to give an ear to my work. His comments and artistic contributions are quintessential. He is not only an accomplished visual artist, a native *congero* but also a wordsmith as well.

Without several other people this book would not be:

Marge Milanese led me through the darkest times an author faces. She epitomizes the spirit of *As Long as You Sing, I'll Dance* and Spontaneous Care Communications with joyfully manifest caring for all. I know she'll take this book in her arms like a newborn, cuddle, coo and praise my dream and even say with an Italian no-nonsense godfather look –"You're sitting on a goldmine. Look at the title alone – who wouldn't want to discuss that?" My friend, Lois Gundrum is to me a practical Joseph, a carpenter who solves all problems. Without Lois, I would not have my refuge and safe place. Both The Legal Project and the Community Loan Fund cleared up much confusion and gave me the green light to go ahead with publishing this book.

Finally, this book is intended as a tribute to the Religious of the Sacred Heart (RSCJ) and their traditions of care, love and contemplative life throughout the world.

When asked how I liked my job as Director of Activities at Kenwood Convent, a Continuing Care Retirement Community, I would often quote poet/artist William Blake: "Gratitude is heaven itself."

I meant that I was so thankful for the daily opportunity to provide programs for these retired Sisters of the Society of the Sacred Heart who expressed endless gratitude and vowed to love and thank me forever through their prayers.

For those of you who tirelessly push dependent elders in wheelchairs to programs and/or taxi seniors to stores, movies or scenic rides, I want to share a personal thank you letter that could help you feel the appreciation that may never be expressed as poetically as in this note from Sr. Mary Raney, RSCJ:

"Dear, dear Julia, None of my many friends have ever drowned for me, never had their beautiful orange dress drenched for me, nor their hair-do quashed flat for me except YOU! How do I begin to say thank you for such kindness…."

This note is written on a card from the Cape Cod cards that Sr. Mary bought for one dollar a box when I drove her through a sudden monsoon to a Christmas Tree Shoppe in Albany. In the same way, spoken and unspoken appreciation from your care partners can help you feel a little heavenly.

Sr. Edna Tierney, RSCJ, was 102 years old when she dictated this grateful note that blesses all the hours and moments we spend at the side of dependent seniors describing the things that they cannot see or hear anymore:

"I appreciate deeply your efforts to 'be my eyes' in your many programs. The last one was a movie 'An Inconvenient Truth.' At that time I also found out that movies are on something called *DVD's* !"

Although I could never answer many of Sr. Tierney's persistent questions such as "Where did they get the stones to build the Appian Way?" she always appreciated my attentive listening.

I have written this book to thank all those who have given me the opportunity to care for them; admittedly, though, with a sly secret hope that others will enjoy caring for me as well.

Julia Soto Lebentritt

Julia's Spontaneous Life

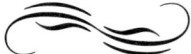

The music of a woodland pond surrounded me as a child on vacations at Dyken Pond. Still there was little concern then for nature, music or a child's amazing growth. Children were not encouraged to be spontaneous and open when I was growing up. Children were seen not heard, although lullabies were sung and stories read to me by my hardworking parents and older brothers and sister. At age 25 suddenly I endured life's real lessons. In the process of recovering from my own near death and after losing my baby, I had a second birth. As I awoke from anesthesia, I found her, this child myself lying in a hospital bed listening to my loved one reading "Winnie The Pooh" to me. Later living in Vermont, I let this child feel free to explore meanings of life and death, studying deep spiritual teachings while climbing green mountains.

Since childhood has been the mission of my life, identifying what a child is, how a child grows, and where we all are children all our lives, needing our childhood affirmed, reenacted and applauded, I am committed to enriching resources for lost childhood.

The musical language of poetry thrives in the nursery. I found my way into the Lower Eastside of Manhattan when I raised my hand to volunteer to do research on lullabies for a music therapy class. The sound of the word alone attracted me. An out-of-print book by Leslie Daiken gave me the idea to include a project in the grant I was writing. "New York City Lullabies" would be field recordings of people singing children to sleep in diverse urban settings and a published 60-minute audiocassette.

I was surprised to find the use of traditional materials in the city environment. My simple idea patterned on Daiken's work in London for the BBC became a reality with the first grant award from New York State Council on the Arts in 1981. I spent long hours with my informants and their children, in bed or wiring bedrooms, and equally long hours alone listening, transcribing and selecting audio and writing journal notes. The project was supervised by consultant Barbara Kirshenblatt-Gimblett, Ph.D. founder/director of New York University Performance Studies Department, and included presentations sponsored by NYU and Columbia University Ethnomusicology Departments in which the lullaby singers demonstrated singing their children to sleep. The perspective I brought to the project as a writer, poet and teacher shaped the many publications, audiovisuals, NPR programs, workshops, presentations and writings that followed. A review by Elizabeth Tucker for *New York Folklore* gave positive commentary and credentials to my work in lullabies:

"From the standpoint of folklore scholarship, this tape accomplishes several missions: clarification of the lullaby as a genre, exploration of an urban multicultural setting and linkage between traditional texts and poetic reflections."

Along the way I kept writing a book about lullabies, one that has shape-shifted several times before my eyes and today exists here.

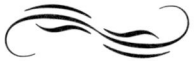

Exploring spontaneity in various art forms made me more aware of what I have discovered about the need for spontaneous communications in our work as caregivers.

Emerging as a woman writer in the 70s, I explored like many other women of my time a newfound freedom to be myself especially in artistic expressions and lifestyle.

Prior to lullaby collecting, as a poet in Connecticut and New York sponsored by state commissions on the arts, I taught poetry in artist residencies at schools. Sound poetry became my vehicle as I sought to bring my love of musical language to more people with a playful collaborative spirit. One day walking on the beach after teaching in the schools, I heard my poetry taking new shapes and sounds, breaking out from the conventional voices I explored. This sound poetry was also performance poetry. I joined with my student poets exploring ways of bringing more of the origins of our texts alive using musical arrangements, spontaneous improvisations, choral readings, drama, dance and accompanying tapes and visuals. As the Director of a Poetry/Theatre/Dance Program at Real Art Ways in Hartford, I was able to bring some of the leading innovative artists including John Cage, The Bread & Puppet Theatre, and Allen Ginsberg to public stages. I also explored authentic movement with Contact Improvisation, a spontaneous style of dance that gives a dancer information by being present.

I chose housing that allowed me to pick up stakes spontaneously and go elsewhere, living in tents on back meadows, seasonal camps on lakes and in artist communities. I followed the ways of Native Americans and older tribal people by living in a remote village in Alaska, then an isolated mountain cabin in northern Vermont, where I encountered paths of action often based on the experience of the moment and fresh insightful immediate solutions like those of a child.

I found teachers, native elders, especially grandmothers in many places who taught me the spontaneous freedom of traditional ways such as, basket weaving, seining, gardening and traveling alone in wilderness. I learned values that the current popular culture did not value – community, presence, respect for all forms of life, living and dead – curative factors that help me deal now with pain, loss, separations, transitions and communications in relationships. All this while I didn't use the word "spontaneous" to describe my life and artistic work but others did.

"What I admire most about New York City Lullabies is its preservation of natural context.... Lullaby singers, found through ads, workshops and performances, welcomed Julia Lebentritt into their homes for recordings of intimate going-to-sleep rituals. The result is a *spontaneous* set of performances that brings lullabies to life for the listener."
>Elizabeth Tucker, *New York Folklore*

"Lebentritt's audiences are happy to rediscover the music of words....On the page too, the poems are lively and raw, retaining the *spontaneous* state of their birth as if refusing to be tamed."
>Marcelle Mekies, *The Hartford Advocate*

"For the concert you were truly a mistress of ceremony. You presided over an event that you made seem both wonderfully warm and *spontaneous*; in it you found the special-ness of each contribution including that of little Darya."
>Leonore Lieblen, Chair of Lullapalooza,
>April 29th Montreal Lullabies 2007

Although I didn't use the word to describe myself, I discovered Spontaneous Care Communications as my soul-driven business name a couple years ago during an intense eight-month-long master's course online taught by writer Isabel Parlett. All my training prior to Isabel's Parlance Training left me talking in other's terminology about my work, using words that end in -er or initials like M.F.A.

Now I feel empowered to guide people to slow down to a speed where life can be lived richly, sensuously, symbolically and lovingly. Isabel's whole brain integrative approach made my mind much less conflicted, more focused, confident and capable of following, controlling and weaving threads of thought into clear patterns.

See Isabel Parlett's website at www.parlancetraining.com.

My writing continues to grow as does my business leaving me with a feeling that my work is essential and a gift. I am thrilled to hear from others about *As Long as You Sing, I'll Dance*. It is my hope that my understanding of the communications needed to discover the joy of connecting more deeply will continue to grow. It is my prayer that science will find healing for this painful and prevalent illness. I encourage others to innovate and share more ways to practice giving and getting care.

Julia Soto Lebentritt
Reciprocal Caregiving Trainings
~Discover the joy of connecting more deeply~
www.reciprocalcare.com
julia@reciprocalcare.com

NOTES

Introductory matter

Abiyoyo: Pete Seeger, *Abiyoyo* (New York: Simon & Schuster Books for Young Readers, 1986). Text copyrights 1963, 1964, 1986).

George Leonard, *The Silent Pulse* (New York: E.P. Dutton, 1978), xii.

"While close I hold thee in my arms": Alma Strettell, ed., *Lullabies of many lands collected and rendered into English verse* (London: George Allen, 1896).

Dan Miller, *No More Dreaded Mondays: Ignite Your Passion – And Other Revolutionary Ways to Discover Your True Calling at Work* (Colorado: WaterBrook Press, 2008), 234.

NEW YORK CITY LULLABIES CD:
http://www.cdbaby.com

Part 1. Following the Thread of Our Mothers' Joyful Caregiving

"The deepest changes may take generations": Mary Catherine Bateson, *Peripheral Visions: Learning along the way* (New York: HarperCollinsPublishers, 1994), 89.

ABAC: Alzheimer's Association, *Activity Based Alzheimer Care: Building a Therapeutic Program* (Illinois: Alzheimer's Disease and Related Disorders Association, Inc., 2000). See http://www.alz.org

"theory of retrogenesis": John Fauber quotes Reisberg: "If caregivers understand that Alzheimer's patients are like regressing children and provide the appropriate care depending on the stage, the descent will be less painful, said Reisberg, a professor of psychiatry and clinical director of the Silberstein Aging & Dementia Center at New York University." John Fauber, "Alzheimer's: Patient, family living life in reverse," *Milwaukee Journal Sentinal*, June 23, 2002.

Psychiatrist Barry Reisberg invented the term "retrogenesis" and first presented it to the International Psychogeriatric Association on August 16, 1999.

Spreading John Zeisel's good news: John Zeisel, Ph.D., *I'm Still Here: A Breakthrough Approach to Understanding Someone Living with Alzheimer's* (New York: Penguin Group, 2009), 56-63.

John Leland, "In 'Sweetie' and 'Dear,' a Hurt for the Elderly," *New York Times Educational Supplement*, Nov. 2, 2008.

"Those ending their lives in the helplessness of old age....": Dr. Paul E. Ruskin, M.D., "We Must Change Our Perspectives," *Journal of the American Medical Association* (1983).

The caregiver's challenge: Carol Bowlby Sifton, *Navigating the Alzheimer's Journey: A Compass For Caregiving* (Baltimore, MD: Health Professions Press, Inc., 2004), 195-197.

Phases of Care: *Roget's International Thesaurus*™ Fourth Edition Revised by Robert L. Chapman (NY: Thomas T. Crowell Company, 1977), 665.

The return to the first language: Carol Bowlby Sifton, *Navigating the Alzheimer's Journey: A Compass For Caregiving*, 195-197.

Mary's Mother: Collected from Mary C. Schaefer, Organizational Development Consultant, President of Artemic Path, LLC. Visit http://www.maryschaefer.com

Part 2. Rhythmic Movements and Spontaneous Songs

Mmmmmmmm – they're all thoughts: Based on Track 3 of the "New York City Lullabies" CD and Song Bank Archives recordings of Robbie McCauley.

"A Patient's Story": Kenneth B. Schwartz, "A Patient's Story." See The Schwartz Center for Compassionate Healthcare. http://www.theschwartzcenter.org

Simple human touch: Federico Garcia Lorca, *Deep Song and Other Prose* (New York: New Directions Publishing Corporation, 1980). Translated and edited by Christopher Maurer.

"These acts of kindness…": Kenneth B. Schwartz, "A Patient's Story."

Finger dancing: Based on the innovative therapeutic work of the Father of the Drum Circle, Arthur Hull, "Circuitry Exercise: The Finger Dance." See Arthur Hull, *Drum Circle Spirit: Facilitating Human Potential Through Rhythm* (Reno, Nevada: White Cliffs Media, Inc. 1998), 61-66.

Connecting the eyes with the ears and the skin: Mary's mother's story collected from Mary C. Schaefer, Organizational Development Consultant, President of Artemic Path, LLC. Visit http://www.maryschaefer.com

Leader's Guide: Harriet the monkey: George B. Schaller, *The Year of the Gorilla* (Chicago: The University of Chicago Press, 1964, 1988).

Helping Hands: See http://www.monkeyhelpers.org

"Generally when threatened or upset…": Peter A. Levine, *In An Unspoken Voice: How the Body Releases Trauma and Restores Goodness* (Berkeley, California: North Atlantic Books, 2012).

"Dance the mother of all dances": Gordon Neufeld, Ph.D., and Gabor Mate, M.D., *Hold On to Your Kids: Why Parents Need to Matter More Than Peers* (New York: Ballantine Books, 2004), 185.

Part 3. Traditions

"Attachment rituals…": Gordon Neufeld, Ph.D., and Gabor Mate, M.D., *Hold On to Your Kids: Why Parents Need to Matter More Than Peers*, 181–182.

Leader's Guide: Praise songs: Leslie Daiken, *The Lullaby Book* (London: Edmund Ward Publishers LTD, 1959), 22.

Leader's Guide: Harvest sensory treasures: Colleen K. Dodt, *The Essential Oils Book* (Pownal, Vermont: Storey Communications, 1996), 135-137.

Nurturing moonlit memories: Ruth Crawford Seeger, *American Folk Songs for Children* (Garden City, New York: Doubleday & Co., 1948), 21.

CODA: "Rest is a communion of love" is a quote from a Mother's Day booklet that I once gave to my mother and found again in her drawer. "Trust – Rest in God" was written by Caryll Houselander (copyright 1956).

"Though shadows dark": Dorothy Berliner Commins, comp., *Lullabies of the World* (New York: Random House, 1967).

Many of these intimate and touching caregiving moments are based on Song Bank Archives recordings, "New York City Lullabies" CD, and the "Lullaby Journal".

I want to acknowledge and thank the adults and children in New York City who allowed me to come into their lives, sometimes homes, sometimes bedrooms and beds, to record and share their lullaby traditions.